Five Elements, Six Conditions

A Taoist Approach to Emotional Healing, Psychology, and Internal Alchemy

Five Elements, Six Conditions

A Taoist Approach to Emotional
Healing, Psychology, and
Internal Alchemy

Gilles Marin

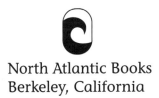

North Atlantic Books
Berkeley, California

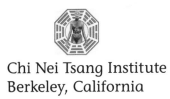

Chi Nei Tsang Institute
Berkeley, California

Published by
North Atlantic Books
P.O. Box 12327
Berkeley, California 94712

Chi Nei Tsang Institute
2812 Telegraph Avenue
Berkeley, California 94705

Cover art by Mouna Ghossoub
Cover design by Jan Camp
Book design by Susan Quasha
Printed in the United States of America

Five Elements, Six Conditions: A Taoist Approach to Emotional Healing, Psychology, and Internal Alchemy is sponsored by the Society for the Study of Native Arts and Sciences, a nonprofit educational corporation whose goals are to develop an educational and crosscultural perspective linking various scientific, social, and artistic fields; to nurture a holistic view of arts, sciences, humanities, and healing; and to publish and distribute literature on the relationship of mind, body, and nature.

North Atlantic Books' publications are available through most bookstores. For further information, call 800-337-2665 or visit our website at www.northatlanticbooks.com.

Substantial discounts on bulk quantities are available to corporations, professional associations, and other organizations. For details and discount information, contact our special sales department.

Library of Congress Cataloging-in-Publication Data

Marin, Gilles.
    Five elements, six conditions : a Taoist approach to emotional healing, psychology, and internal alchemy / by Gilles Marin.
            p. ; cm.
    Includes bibliographical references and index.
    ISBN-13: 978-1-55643-593-5 (trade paper)
    ISBN-10: 1-55643-593-2 (trade paper)
    1. Qi gong. 2. Medicine, Chinese. 3. Massage therapy. 4. Taoism. I. Society for the Study of Native Arts and Sciences. II. Title.
    [DNLM: 1. Complementary Therapies. 2. Medicine, Chinese Traditional. 3. Mental Healing. 4. Mind-Body Relations (Metaphysics) 5. Qi. WB 890 M337f 2006]
    RM727.C54M37 2006
    615.8'52—dc22
                                        2006009465

1 2 3 4 5 6 7 8 9 UNITED 12 11 10 09 08 07 06

To Emily and Jesse, and to the Power that brings people together.

Contents

Illustrations

Chi-Kung and Meditations

Acknowledgments

First and foremost, I would like to thank my clients and students for their trust and courage in helping to provide the material to write this book.

My heartfelt thanks go out to numerous teachers for their patience and guidance, especially Master Mantak Chia for bringing Chi Nei Tsang out of the esoteric world and into daily reality, and for his teachings on Taoist Chi-Kung and functional meditations. My deepest appreciation to Dr. Stephen T. Chang for his extremely wide spectrum of teaching the Five Elements, Classical Chinese Medicine, Feng Shui, and the I'Ching. To my friend Juan Li for his enlightened perspective on the I'Ching—I am looking forward to his work being published.

My extreme gratitude goes to Francesca Fasano for editing my broken English, for her sharp eye and excellent suggestions throughout the book, and to my publishers, Richard Grossinger and Lindy Hough, and their fine team at North Atlantic Books.

My heartfelt gratitude goes to Master Kazuaki Tanahashi for his magnificent calligraphy, and to my friend Mouna Ghossoub for her exquisite artwork.

I would also like to acknowledge my good friend Stephanie Wilger for her emotional support, by assisting me, teaching, and giving treatments during the writing of this book. My greatest appreciation goes to Stephanie Peters, Maureen Davison, Francesca Fasano, and all of my assistants at the Chi Nei Tsang Institute for their support and dedication to making sure that things got done.

Warm thanks to my friend Kurt Miller for sharing his knowledge on the Feldenkrais method and for keeping me in shape and out of pain with regular treatments, and to Isabelle Pelaud and Simon Ho, for their friendship, moral support, and networking help.

And last but not least, thank you from the bottom of my heart to all my teaching assistants for carrying on the flag, and to all the friends of Chi Nei Tsang, who have participated in developing and promoting Chi Nei Tsang and healing from within.

Preface

This book is for anyone interested in understanding the work of healing at the physical as well as the mental, emotional, and spiritual levels. To understand healing at these multiple levels, we need to use a mental process that allows us to have a global appreciation of these different levels of existence. This is why I find it necessary to use the Eastern concept of the Taoist Law of the Five Elemental Forces of Nature.

To be complete, any healing method needs to embody a holistic perspective on health and existence. And to be accepted by the general public, it also has to make sense. In addition, I believe that human consciousness has reached a level that requires clarity rather than mysticism. We no longer live in a time when it was enough for us to just "believe," to have blind faith in our doctors and other health care providers, or our religious leaders, for that matter. I chose the Taoist approach because of its comprehensive cosmology, scientific soundness, and use of the Law of Five Elemental Forces of Nature (also called the Law of the Five Elements or Law of Five Phases)—and because it has a universal grasp of life. Its origins are deeply rooted in Taoist esoteric monastic practices and traditional wisdom, and it has survived the test of time. Today, despite the global pervasiveness of conventional allopathic medicine, it is the most popular traditional medical method used among Asian populations. In the West it has become a way of thinking that reconciles the most current scientific perspectives with both ancient and traditional philosophy and cosmology. Taoism's description of the world integrates completely with the most up-to-date theories in modern physics. Taoist cosmology, with its system of polarity (Yin and Yang), its Five Elemental Forces, and its sixty-four binary representations (I'Ching), is still, to this day, the most accurate and dynamic representation of existence. It has been used by scientists all over the world to help them progress in their methods of research, and many have written books about modern discoveries proving the truth of Taoist wisdom.[1]

This book is based on more than twenty years of clinical practice and personal experience in a Taoist method of healing called Chi Nei Tsang, along with the exploration of a very wide spectrum of healing techniques as a client and practitioner of massage therapy. It is also the fruit of a regular practice of martial arts such as Aikido and T'ai-Chi-Chuan, different forms of Chi-Kung *(qigong),* and various Taoist meditations since my first involvement with Aikido, bio-energy, and massage therapy in the mid-seventies when I was still a teenager. I owe my understanding of the working of the Taoist system of the Five Elemental Forces of Nature primarily to two great Taoist teachers, Dr. Stephen T. Chang and Master Mantak Chia. Dr. Chang taught me the principles of classical Traditional Chinese Medicine, acupuncture, internal exercises (Chi-Kung), classical Chinese herbology, the I'Ching, Feng-Shui, and Taoist philosophy. Master Chia has been my mentor in esoteric Taoist meditations and Chi-Kung practices since my mid-twenties.

It is important to understand that the teachings in this book are not based on particular dogma. They have all been passed down from my mentors, based on practical experience, and have been personally updated from daily learning and personal discovery. This is what I believe to be "true" Taoism, the progressive rediscovery of the right way (Tao) to do things as new events and updated information unfold into history. This tradition has been honored for millennia and passed down directly from masters to students. In China, it gave birth to acupuncture, the use of powerful traditional herbal combinations, and different schools of internal energy exercises and martial arts called Kung-Fu (mastery of a skill), Chi-Kung or Nei-Kung (mastery of Chi and internal processes), and T'ai-Chi-Chuan. It is also at the origin of traditional Chinese sacred architecture and geomancy called Feng-Shui, and of Chi Nei Tsang, the art of internal healing through applied Chi-Kung.

When I began studying Traditional Chinese Medicine, I was both startled and confused by the discrepancies and the many different systems conceived by different doctors, true erudites and authorities in their fields, who seemed at times to contradict one another. Only a long practice of meditation and Chi-Kung revealed the answer to me:

No one is wrong, and everyone is right (from his own perspective). This doesn't mean, however, that everyone's way of doing things will work for me, or for anyone else for that matter. Especially with regard to health, there is only one reality about the truth: Everything is relative. The truth changes according to where we stand. Like every doctor in that tradition, I had to study, investigate, and make sense of all these theories for myself before I could expect results in my own private practice. Therefore, the information contained in this book is not to be taken as dogma. Rather, it is meant to perpetuate a tradition of the search for truth and meaning from a personal and authentic perspective dear to all Taoist scholars and practitioners for millennia. It is designed to teach "how to learn" rather than "what to remember." So don't believe anything written in this book until it makes sense to you in a way that's practical and useful, until you have accepted its truth as your own.

To this effect, after each "lecture," in each chapter, there are specific exercises designed to help you understand and integrate the principles outlined in this book at a more physical level. This is the way I teach at the Chi Nei Tsang Institute and at other centers where these classes are offered. I will not teach any healing techniques without teaching the principles that allowed their discovery. These principles are found in each exercise, meditation, and visualization in this book. These exercises and meditations are drawn from esoteric classical formulas that took several generations to refine and clarify, and have been updated to adapt to the needs of our times. The exercises and meditations follow a progression of difficulty that needs to be respected in order to achieve better results. As with the practices contained in my first book, *Healing from Within with Chi Nei Tsang,* I recommend that you play with them. Don't be too rigid; go for what feels right for you. Every morning choose "something" that feels right, and make it a daily routine to do twenty minutes of this "something" every day. Build your own practice even if you don't have the opportunity to live near a Chi Nei Tsang center where you can join a study group. You don't need to work too hard; all you need is to be steady and regular. Remember that it takes effort to be fully human. Without this kind of discipline, we will not evolve to our full human potential.

Meditation usually takes a lot of training and dedication, with directed guidance. However, meditations and Chi-Kung are not meant to make you do anything unnatural. Every single practice involves nothing more than to be aware of something that is already happening naturally. You need to enhance your awareness to be able to control these natural processes of life a little better, instead of being completely controlled by them. The practices described in this book are adapted to bring even absolute beginners to great insights. For adepts of advanced forms of meditation, you will also find that, in applying these principles, your regular routines will be greatly enhanced. These meditations and exercises are extremely powerful. When practiced regularly from the heart, they will bring you to the highest levels of spiritual practice and add clarity, wisdom, and guidance to your daily life. Many monks and nuns have devoted their lifetimes in monasteries to learning only bits and pieces of these practices, in anonymous seclusion. Please practice with diligence and high spirit out of respect and gratitude for their memories.

Note that in this book I choose to use formal English rather than the commonly adopted Romanized writing of Chinese ideographs (*Chi* and *Chi-Kung*, rather than *qi* and *qigong*). Concept names are capitalized (Chi, Chakra, Liver, Spleen-Pancreas) and shouldn't be mistaken for their English homonyms: for example, Liver means "the energetic system of the Yin Wood function" and is not only the anatomical organ liver, even though the Liver encompasses certain functions of the liver.

When reading this book, you might feel that I am negating both conventional medicine and psychotherapy. Actually, some of my best friends are medical doctors and psychotherapists, and I am very thankful for their knowledge and advice. As I have already stated in *Healing from Within with Chi Nei Tsang*, there is a need for the whole spectrum of healing in the health care community. We actually need more science, not less! Medical and scientific research over the past ten to twenty years has been responsible for many important discoveries. It is the synthesizing work of healing that has been mostly misunderstood and underdeveloped because of its tendency to shroud itself under a thick layer of mysticism. This book is an attempt to lift this mystical shroud, and to make healing more commonly understood, and less disregarded, by the scientific community and the general public, so that healing can be used to make science, in general, and medicine, in particular, more efficient and more human.

Gilles Marin

Whispering Pines, California,

December 2001

There is no intelligence required for healing. To heal, we don't need to be intelligent, we don't need to be good, and we don't need to deserve it. Healing is pure grace. To heal, we do need honesty. We need to be true to ourselves. We need to be able to admit that we have feelings we wish we didn't have. We need to own these feelings so we can outgrow them, and so we can mature as human beings.

G. M.

PART ★ I

Healing and the Universal Laws of Nature

CHAPTER ⭐ 1

Introduction to the Concepts of Healing, Taoism, and Chi Nei Tsang

Five Realizations About Emotional Healing

During my practice of massage therapy and Chi Nei Tsang, my clients regularly tell me how their treatments allow them to make major breakthroughs in their emotional life, and how their physical health improvement brings corresponding mental and emotional transformations. Some of them are amazed at how much their behavior and personality change during the brief period of time that they have experienced Chi Nei Tsang, compared to the length of treatment typically required with psychotherapy.

From a personal point of view, my studies of psychology and my own extended experience with psychotherapy as a client, at best, never really afforded me more than a certain degree of mental satisfaction and awareness about things that need to change, but no satisfying method to effect those changes. Actually, very little deep personal transformation spontaneously emerged from these studies and consultations. No matter how much I understood why I felt a certain way, I would still feel the same or even worse. All this led me to believe that something fundamental was missing from the current psychological approach. Instead of helping us to discover why we feel a certain way and how we become fixated on this, a well-understood healing process should bring us to a place where we can say that we used to feel that way, but that we no longer do.

Considering the poor understanding of the concept of healing and holism in our Western society, the current practices of psychotherapy and psychiatry have very little choice but to be medically oriented and aimed at problem solving. Instead, they should provide the means and support required for healthy growth, constant life enhancement, and spiritual self-guidance—the necessities for outgrowing the inevitable mental crises and emotional distress of modern life, and the frightening mental symptoms that often accompany such crises and stress. This has led me to five essential realizations about emotional healing:

- First, in healing, *we cannot separate the mind from the body.* Each symptom, mental or physical, has a meaning. This meaning reflects the way we generally feel and is always emotionally charged. Different symptoms usually keep repeating the same meaning, so multiple symptoms in us are *always* emotionally related.

- Second, unlike thoughts, *emotions are not rational.* Therefore, they cannot be solved. Besides, we don't choose our feelings; we get them. We don't solve emotional charges; we outgrow them. To outgrow them requires digesting them. We literally grow out of our emotions—we take what we need from them and eliminate what we don't need. Taking what we need makes us stronger, more sensitive, and allows us to expand our awareness further, to feel more and emotionally digest more, to grow even more emotionally mature, and thus more emotionally perceptive.

- Third, *emotions are carried in our bodies as energetic charges that need to be processed physically.* They manifest in significant locations in bodily structures such as joints and muscle groups, to be expressed by bodily attitudes. These energetic charges require digestion and their level of processing can be traced throughout the length of our digestive system.

- Fourth, *the healing process can take place only when there is a chance to recover and awareness is present.* The key to the healing process is awareness, which is always proportional to power and maturity. We possess a failsafe that prevents us from feeling too much when we don't have a sufficient support system, or sufficient maturity or power. This is our protective denial system, our "guardian." It is usually easier to endure pain at the strictly physical level than at the mental-emotional level. Therefore, the evolution of symptomatic responses starts with physical distress, and when a mental connection is made, and the pain is felt at the emotional level, then the physical pain disappears.

• Fifth, *spirit rules healing*. Spirit means guidance and being connected with our reason for being alive. Getting in touch with our life purpose and its enjoyment allows us to adjust our lifestyle, and accept and adapt to necessary changes.

Differentiating Thoughts from Emotions

The primary focus of this book is on emotional healing. To really understand healing means to understand that there is no difference whatsoever between physical, mental, and emotional healing. Emotions are a part of us that we are not accustomed to understanding. In our culture, it is not common practice to sit down and contemplate the world of feelings in a group setting. Even though many of us do this individually as a matter of habit, it is not something that our culture favors outside of a professional setting such as in psychotherapy, or in art and entertainment, which even then have a tendency to be artificial and heavily tainted with a profit-making or propagandist agenda.

Emotions must first be differentiated from thoughts. Thoughts are rational. Thinking uses logic, and belongs to time and space with a linear structure of past, present, and future. Thinking is for problem solving. Thoughts are the product of the frontal lobe of our cerebral cortex—the most advanced part of our nervous system, the most advanced feature in primates, and the latest upgrade in the evolutionary chain. It is so advanced that it doesn't really work at full capacity yet. Scientific research has demonstrated that even the most educated, cultured, literate, well-traveled, and sophisticated among us are using no more than 10 to 15 percent of full capacity, and with constant effort at that. If we relate our humanity to our capacity to use our thinking process, our rationality, and clarity of mind, it means that it takes great effort to be fully human. Being fully human doesn't come naturally to us yet, and it requires a lot of work and cultivation. Even if we understand this principle of mental evolution, new ideas traditionally and systematically get rejected: the time of Galileo and the Inquisition occurred less than 300 years ago, and yet various forms of inquisition still exist today in many so-called intellectual circles. This means that new, unfamiliar ideas, no matter how accurate they are, will feel wrong to most of us.

As for emotions, we have such a difficult time with them that I believe we are still in the dark. Before modern times, emotional research and introspection had always been the domain of the occult, or the spiritual, of the monastic practices and of hermits. Only recently, during the past eighty years of Western civilization, have we attempted to explore a contested scientific approach to human behavior and the reasons for such through the study of psychology. Emotions are nonrational. They are not to be confused with thoughts. They are pure abstraction, and therefore, richer, more complete, and more exacting than thoughts. They come from various parts of our nervous system that work at 100 percent of their capacity at all times. Our emotions are also strongly supported by our endocrine system, which governs our nervous system through hormones such as serotonin, insulin, and adrenaline. Emotions are therefore longer lasting, much faster, and more powerful than thoughts. Unlike our thoughts, we don't choose our emotions; we get them. They don't belong to time or space, to past or future; they only belong to the present, the here and now.

But what are emotions, really? We know that they manifest somatically, and that their manifestation spreads through the whole self. Emotions are felt, so they are also often called feelings. Emotions are truly responsible for behavior. We don't act according to the way we think; we act according to the way we feel. It doesn't matter if we know what is better for us. If we don't ultimately feel like doing something, we won't. Most of the time, our way of thinking is quite powerless when confronted with contradictory feelings. This reflects the biggest crisis of our time: being unable to do what our best knowledge advises us to do. Its influence is far-reaching at all levels of life from communication to relationship, from sports to show business, from education to engineering, and from politics and social studies to law and justice. "What feels right," with all the abstract and irrational content of what "what feels right" means, will always ultimately rule over reason.

We feel with our entire being—body, as well as mind and spirit. When we feel happy, we don't only feel it in our mind and our nervous system. Our face is happy, our heart is happy, our skin, stomach, and even our hair manifest that happiness. When we are sad, our whole body is sad. Feelings carry through our whole body and manifest through what are called *emotional charges,* pockets of energy containing information— what we call *Chi* in Traditional Chinese Medicine. Emotions are carried through our nervous system and our endocrine system. In biology, the endocrine system has a prevalent function of intercellular communication throughout the body, and there are indeed many correlations between what we know of the endocrine system, and the *Chakras,* or energetic-informational centers of the body from Eastern traditions.

Unlike the thoughts, emotions don't care about solutions or comprehension. Understanding them doesn't change them. We can't change feelings the way we do thoughts by "knowing better." The only thing we can do to change our emotions is to outgrow them. This is literal: Emotionally growing means growing physically by digesting these emotions, taking what we need from them, and eliminating what we don't.

Emotions Are the Food of Our Soul

My studies in healing and my practice of Taoist meditation have led me to believe that emotions are the food of our soul. When we talk about "growing" as a person, I understand it literally. We feed every day on different kinds of emotions, and we literally digest them. This makes us grow. Emotional maturity thus means having digested a sufficiently wide spectrum of basic human feelings to allow us to function independent of any form of parental protection, authority figure, or external guidance.

Every day we absorb a certain quantity of emotions in the form of energetic charges created by our body's reactions to feelings. Some of these charges are easy to digest, some harder to digest, and some are quite indigestible. We call these latter type toxic or negative emotions. Where do these charges go when not digested? To exactly the same place that any toxic food would go in our body, to various places of storage: the liver, body fat, the lymphatic system, and any tissue and location that has meaning for that particular charge. Every part of the body has a function, which has a corresponding meaning for the emotional self that is going to hold and hide the charge there.

How can we hide anything inside our own body? We do it all the time, and very easily. All it takes for us not to know anything about ourselves is to make sure communication doesn't reach specific places. Actually, the body can't really forget anything. Unlike the nervous system, which has to constantly select from all the information needed at one time to fit it on the small screen of our awareness, every single cell in our body contains all of the information from all of evolution since the day of creation. So our body doesn't really forget anything; rather, it chooses not to remember something in particular.

We are born to enjoy life. Unfortunately, life is not always enjoyable. To protect us from the horror of emotional distress, our bodies are equipped with a very sophisticated protection system. This denial system protects us from permanently feeling bad from the emotions we don't have the capacity to address due to lack of maturity or knowledge, or a weakness in our support system. This *denial system,* the "guardian," is in charge of hiding the emotions until we are able to meet the conditions that will allow us to digest them and grow from them. Since we are born to enjoy life, every single part of our body is entitled to participate in this enjoyment. When we hide an emotional charge somewhere in our body, this place doesn't feel bad because it has become numb. But, by the same token, it can't feel good either. The role of our guardian is also to let us know when we finally meet the requirements to be able to face our emotions. Once we are mature enough, stable enough, strong enough, and have a sufficient support system, the guardian lets us know this through a symptom. A symptom is then an attempt from our deeper inner self to let us know that it is time to change, time to grow, time to heal.

The main vehicles for communication in the body are the nervous and endocrine systems, while the principal modes of communication are contact and movement. The nerves have to make contact in order to carry information because they have to carry the impulse, the energy that carries information. Unlike electricity that runs through inanimate matter, the energy running through a live body, Chi, follows different rules: It needs movement to carry on. The mode of movement through our body is our breath. It is our breath that pumps oxygen in our chest and it is the cellular breath that makes sure that the product of breath, the spark of life, is evenly distributed to every tissue and cell in our bodies. It is well recognized in Traditional Chinese Medicine that our breath carries our Chi, that spark of life that carries the energy and the information of life at all levels in our body and allows us to feel inner movement.

Our breath is the inner bridge that connects all levels of awareness within us. Not to feel a certain place in our body requires not breathing there. We stop breathing there so we stop feeling it. It numbs, and becomes able to hold any amount of tension without our feeling it. This is the reason we can go through our whole life with unnoticed muscular contractions in our shoulders, for example, or in our neck or our back that we would not be able to tolerate if we were actually made to feel them. When we are made aware of such contractions through exercise, yoga, or a massage therapy session, it usually comes out either as a pain, or as what we call a "healing crisis" when it expresses itself as a symptom. It takes a tremendous amount of effort for us to keep our body out of alignment. If we choose to do it so systematically, we must have good reason. It is easier to endure pain at the physical level than to experience it at the emotional level!

Hidden emotional charges explain the reasons we have a hard time recovering after a minor accident. Strictly physical problems go away quickly. If they don't, it is because there are hidden charges creating a physical, energetic, and informational blockage that prevents us from recovering. Osteoporosis is a good example of chronically hidden emotional charges. Working with osteoporosis clients, one learns that not all the bones in their body are affected the same way. Some bones are not affected at all, and the bones that are affected are not necessarily the ones that succumb to weakness due to non-use. This is because the site of most weakness in the bones always relates to places of chronic contractions, of which the client is unaware or where the client is unable to relax (typically, jaws, different parts of the spine, hips, shoulders, or neck). The muscles in constant contraction leach more calcium from the local bones, and prevent these bones from regenerating at the normal rate. When an osteoporosis client releases the charge from that location and allows the muscles there to relax and be healthy, the bones in that particular location improve dramatically.[2] Of course, hormones also play a major role there. They have to in order to support the strategy of the emotional body in hiding chronic patterns of tension (see Chapter 5).

We carry some of these emotional charges for years, even for generations when they are passed down through patterns of habit. In *Healing from Within with Chi Nei Tsang* (hereinafter referred to simply as *Healing from Within*), we explored the digestive aspects of these emotional charges. In this book, we explore the conditions by which such digestion is possible, how the different stages of that digestion are expressed, and how we can actually map out the manifestation of these different emotional charges throughout our entire body. Once we understand how our body deals with this, then we practice the Fusion of the Five Elemental Forces meditation (see Chapter 7). This meditation uses a formula that has been practiced and refined for hundreds of years in the spiritual disciplines of the East to help our entire mind, not only our thinking mind, to process and grow from the experience of emotional digestion. This formula is based on working with the Five Elemental Forces of Nature to find harmony within and outside us in this ever-expanding universe.

What Is Healing?

First, we must define "healing." The conventional medical approach is to cure symptoms and conditions that cause suffering through the use of synthesized drugs, surgery, and, more recently, genetic engineering. The basic philosophy behind this approach is the assumption that nature is not to be trusted—that nature has problems that need to be solved through human intervention.

The holistic approach, on the other hand, assumes that since we are the product of millions of years of evolution, and since we are still in the gene pool, we are pretty much perfect, at least to the degree of perfection possible in a universe in constant evolution. Perfection, as a matter of fact, is not an attribute of nature; therefore, it is not a human attribute either. What is natural and human is to be able to improve all the time. It is to progress constantly, following the need to adapt to the ever-changing, ever-evolving world. Something perfect cannot be ameliorated any further. Perfection is not an attribute of this universe; it is an attribute of what rules the universe. If we experience diseases and conditions, it is either as an attempt to adapt or because we lack the information that would either protect us from or prevent these health problems. Symptoms are usually messages from within, asking for help and demanding evolution. Most of our pains come from healthy reactions to unhealthy situations in our bodies in which we often find ourselves involved.

The principle of health—what is healthy—draws a very fine line between too much and not enough. Health is not about balance since life is about motion and movement. Complete balance describes a static world not even found in death. To live well, we need a constant state of imbalance that moves us in the direction of the progression, evolution, and expansion of the universe to maintain harmony within it. Too little would require the constant effort of having to catch up with the pace of life, while too much would bring us ahead of our time with the catastrophic results of non-adaptation and rejection. Indeed, humanity, throughout all civilizations, has always experienced this full spectrum.

Healing is also about fulfilling our life purpose. It involves being in harmony with the evolution of our time. Our life purpose is about fulfilling our individual role as a member of existence. We come into life inheriting a universe that is complete. This heritage is biological, historical, geographical, cultural, ethnic, and ecological, and it encompasses the physical, mental, emotional, and spiritual aspects of the self. Many of us get sick from "not being on the right track." We find ourselves in life situations that are foreign to our nature or unfair to our spirit, and we find our bodies and souls rebelling against this. Most of the time, our conscious mind is oblivious to the situation, and, only after enduring systemic symptoms, are we given the chance to make the necessary changes to go through our healing process.

The Healing Process

The healing process is the physical and/or mental manifestation of the internal conflict between the part of us that wants to evolve and grow, and the part of us that is afraid of going through the pains of change and growth. Change is the hardest thing to go through in life and requires the transition time of the healing process, which often necessitates the intervention of symptoms, accidents, or life crises to bring awareness of the need for change.

The healing process is, thus, the often-uncomfortable transition time between that place of familiarity we all come from, and that new better place, which is still not familiar enough to be comfortable. This is why the healing process is often called a healing crisis. Healing is always a step forward in evolution. There is no healing without change. Once we are healed, there is no turning back and no suffering through the same symptoms again. The healing process does not need to be painful, but will always contain a large amount of confusion where the old patterns, the old frame of reference, the old self, need to be discarded. For this reason, specific conditions have to be met in order for healing to take place (see Chapter 8).

Emotional Release: The First Law of Thermodynamics Applied to Psychotherapy

While traveling through Polynesia and Hawaii searching for peace and quiet to work on my books and guided meditations, I learned a lot by being in contact with native Polynesians and by observing the reactions of Westerners to the natives' way of life. Hygiene is a big issue on the islands. Dwellings are traditionally spotless and elevated from the ground, and shoes are kept outdoors. But what horrifies the non-locals is the amount of trash left on beaches where the local people live. Natives have been using these beaches for thousands of years, living, eating, fishing, surfing, sleeping, and enjoying life there. Everything they use—plant leaves to wrap and cook their food, coconut shells, bones, sea shells, and leftovers from cooking—is organic, biodegradable, and part of the eternal recycling aspect of nature and their island. Such detritus wouldn't remain on the beach any longer than the next tide, and, in any case, no longer than a night or two before starting to decompose. By the end of the week, everything would return to the continuing decomposition-recomposition cycle of life and death. To the indigenous mind, there is no such thing as dumping, especially on a small island. In fact, the very idea of trash and dumping is considered extremely disrespectful. Everything has its place and order. The locals often say jokingly when people don't tidy up, "Please clean up after yourself, your mother doesn't work here!"—meaning that whatever you dump, someone else has to pick up.

Indigenous habits didn't change readily with the advent of plastic, canning, and packaging. The natives have no concept of something that is so durable and dirty that you have to "make it disappear by hiding it," even in the face of the tropical sun and the mighty Pacific Ocean. Does anything like this really exist? What is this Western concept of dumping, anyway? Does anything we dump ever disappear? Well, nothing disappears. This is the law of thermodynamics in modern physics where only two things exist, energy and information: "Nothing is created, nothing disappears; energy is either transmitted or transformed." We are so used to "disposing" of garbage that we have a tendency to think that when we take the garbage "out" at night, and it is "gone" in the morning, it is just another commodity of the civilized world such as starting a car, using a computer, and buying groceries at the store. We don't need to know how these machines operate, and how they are built, or who grows the vegetables, and how they got to the store. Likewise, we don't need to worry about dumping. "It is taken care of ..."—or is it?

From the psychological perspective, there is no real dumping either, in the true sense of the word. There is no such thing as a final emotional release. When we release emotionally, an energetic charge is moving, changing place, perhaps changing shape, but it is *not* disappearing. It is moving, it is transforming. It is a process. When we become aware of an emotional charge and feel it stirring, it doesn't mean that it has been taken care of even if we cry, jump, scream, or go into convulsion and spasm. Such actions are mere reactions to an unpleasant situation. They don't mean, in any way, that the work of healing is complete.

Again, whatever we dump has to be picked up by someone else, and, at the emotional level, we all dump and pick up and dump some more. Emotional charges are dumped and picked up and dumped again and again until they find a place of transformation, until they get recycled and put to use again. In the meantime, dumped emotional charges haunt the places where they were released and affect us like a parasite wavelength affects reception in a radio or a cordless telephone. This is what we feel when we walk into a place where there has been a heated argument, or a psychotherapy treatment room after a session. This is the "charged atmosphere" in a courtroom or a stadium. Since emotional charges also get released in people, this has a big impact on the quality of relationship we have with others. This is why it is important to do Chi-Kung and meditation to change the energy of the environment into a more positive and more loving atmosphere.

Real emotional processing is an emotional transformation that changes the negative aspects of the charge into positive ones. This happens with a shift in the whole person, not only at the emotional level, but also at the physical, mental, and spiritual levels. There is no such thing as changing only here and there. The body is very consistent: If one part of us changes, not only the whole body, but our whole personality has to shift and adapt to that change. It is not a part of our body, or our mind, or a part of our emotional makeup changing. It is we in that part of our body, we in that part of our mind, we in that part of our emotional self who change. In short, our whole being changes.

When such a change occurs, it is by using the same biological matter, the same energy that has been there all along. Only now it has been recycled and digested, and it has transformed and evolved. This recycling aspect of emotional energy is a very important one. Chi is like water. When water circulates, oxygen enters the water and kills bacteria. When water stagnates, bacteria proliferate, and the water becomes poisonous. Like water, when Chi circulates, it is healthy. When it slows down and stops, it becomes toxic. We should never store Chi for very long. When we "store" Chi during certain Chi-Kung exercises, it is only for a short time, the same way we store air in a bagpipe to play it, or water in a tank for constant use in a house. The air and water stored there are never the same because they keep circulating.

Our work as practitioners is not only to merely dislodge the emotional charge, but it is also to make sure that the energy contained there is going to move and change. There is no point in moving dirt from under one carpet to under another one. But neither can we "dump" that dirt, even to put it under a cosmic size carpet! That dirt has to be put back to use. Life has to be put back into it, then it has to be put in a place where it can be enjoyed. This is what happens during healing: The energy spent to hold a pathology in place turns into the healing surge that melts tumors and reverses diseases, and the negative emotional pattern turns into a positive one. No energy is lost, no energy is gained. This is the law of physics, the law of nature.

Extraordinary Chi

In *Healing from Within,* we explored the concept of Chi as energy pregnant with information, and the inseparability of energy from the information that it holds. Chi feeds the various functions in the body; it thus takes on the qualities of these functions. When the Chi goes through our Heart and endocrine system (Heart Controller) in our blood, it becomes Fire Chi; when going through the Kidneys and our genes, it becomes Water Chi; in our Spleen-Pancreas, digestive system, and muscles, it is Earth Chi; in our Liver and nervous system, it becomes Wood Chi; and in our Lungs and skin, it is Metal Chi. The energy and information that constitute our Chi is subject to improvement through learning and self-cultivation. When applied to a skill, it is called Kung-Fu, and when applied to health, Chi-Kung.

In this book, we are emphasizing the most classical aspect of Chi brought about by its very etymology. The classical Chinese character for Chi is composed of two ideographs: the first on the top, formally written in four strokes, represents a flow meaning "air," "vapor," or "breath," which we translate as flow of breath (see Figure 1),[3] and the second ideograph, on the bottom, formally written in six strokes, representing the notion of "rice," as well as "essence." The rice ideograph symbolizes the presence of the life force, the energy contained in every grain of rice. It is the spark of life. Together these two ideographs represent the flow of the life force, the energy and the information that brings life. Chi is therefore not neutral. Chi is the energy carrying the deliberate intent to promote life and existence. It is a power that comes with an intention. It is the breath of creation. For this reason, Chi is often translated as "the breath of God." It is then understandable why the essentially atheist Chinese Communist ideology chose to "simplify" the character Chi by removing the "spark of life contained in a single grain of rice" ideograph, keeping only the "flow of breath" ideograph, thereby eliminating any spiritual connection with the concept of Chi and translating it as the neutral concept of energy or breath. (See Figure 1 for ideographs of classical Chi.[4])

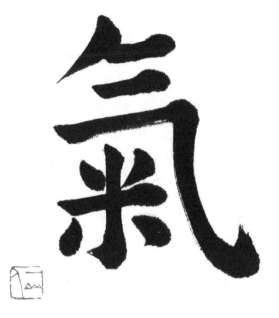

Classical Chi
The breath of life

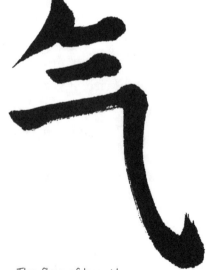

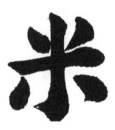

The spark of life within a grain of rice

The flow of breath
Chi in modern Chinese

Figure 1.
Ideographs of
classical Chi

Four ways to write Chi (Ki) by Master Kazuaki Tanahashi

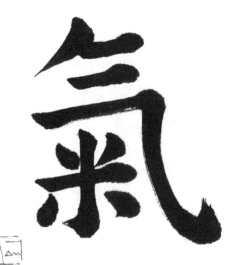

Formal in ten strokes

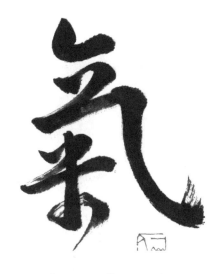

Cursive in four strokes

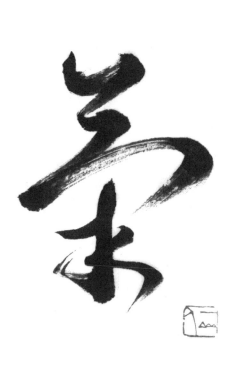

Two strokes

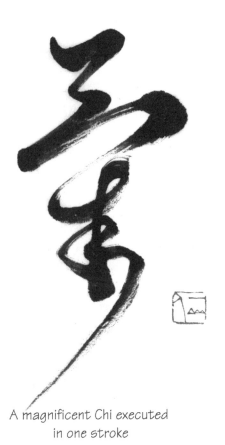

A magnificent Chi executed
in one stroke

Figure 2.
Four ways to
write Chi

In medicine, Chi is used to establish the changes that bring healing. When used in martial arts to kill or in situations where life is no longer tolerable, Chi ultimately effects the changes that renew existence. The quality of the Chi establishes the power delivered by the level of consciousness: If the energy is corrupted or somewhat deficient, it results in a negative charge, as disease or suffering. If the energy is healthy and abundant, it promotes good health and happiness, and the development of human consciousness. Power and consciousness come with responsibilities, which are ultimately aimed at protecting and promoting quality of life and health.

Because of its extensive use of Chi (Ki in Japanese), the martial art Aikido is so powerful that, to this day, it can't be safely used in competition. It has been called the ultimate martial art, the last of a long lineage of Budo, the Japanese martial tradition. Morhie Ueshiba (1883–1969), the founder of Aikido, was probably the last of the Japanese "invincible warriors."[5] However, like legendary warriors Myamoto Musashi, author of *The Book of Five Rings,* and, before him, General Sun Tzu, author of *The Art of War,* Ueshiba spent his life promoting peace and nonviolence. Furthermore, Ueshiba was the first to introduce the concept of "protecting the enemy," the ultimate art of diplomacy, the art of the peace warrior. By protecting the enemy, we outgrow our bestiality and protect our humanity. There are then no losers, only winners. Aikido—Ai for "togetherness," Ki (Chi) for "life force," and Do (Tao) for "the way"—translates as "the way of harmony." Martial art, at this level of consciousness, then becomes the art of winning rather than the art of fighting, with the connotation of winning over, not defeating, the "enemy."

Why a Taoist Approach?

There are three main reasons, as outlined below.

First, we need a *methodology for treatments.*

We need a clear methodology, a good system to help support clients in the midst of their processes. Healing generally happens in several waves. There is the immediate wave that comes out of the treatment, and there are also the long-term, long-range waves that lie beneath the surface, which can take several days, weeks, months, or longer to find the opportunity to emerge with their transformational effects. Clients need to be told of the possible reactions they might expect so that they will recognize them and validate them when they happen, and so that they won't come out of their healing process because of fear. They are not becoming worse; they are becoming aware! This is the time for introspection and patience, not the time for panic and rushing to the emergency room or the medicine cabinet. Medical doctors have to be able to recognize the healing process so that they do not unwittingly do something irreversible with emergency procedures.

Second, we need a *sound philosophy of life and existence to support healing.*

When we heal, we change. Our behavior changes, our reactions change, and our tastes change. These changes can occur in a very predictable way for someone who has studied the Tao, the way things have a tendency to change according to the Taoist wisdom of the Five Elemental Forces of Nature and the I'Ching. These natural tendencies were discovered long ago through systematic observation of nature and its fundamental energies.

Modern physics has taught us about the four forces that simultaneously tend to cause the motion of a body and hold our planet together: the gravitational force, the electromagnetic force, and the strong and weak nuclear forces. There are also forces of a different nature that allow life to take place. These forces are associated with essential elements or tendencies, as opposed to the chemical elements found in the periodic table. Because of their relationship to life and the manifestations of life, these elemental forces are often referred to as alchemical forces, to distinguish them from the inert chemicals found in the composition of nature.

In order to have life, these five alchemical forces must work in harmony. They represent the nature of everything alive and are the direct result of the manifestation of our universe, called Tai-Chi, the "Great Universe," the universe of polarities, of dimensions and oppositions, and of time and space.

Briefly stated, these five elemental forces are:

• Fire, for maximum expansion, substantiality, and heat, ruling the southern direction

- Water, for maximum contraction, essential qualities, and cold, ruling the northern direction
- Wood, for whatever is warming, expanding, and growing, ruling the East, the direction of the sunrise
- Metal, for whatever is cooling, condensing, and reflecting, ruling the West, the direction of the sunset
- Earth, for the harmonizing, nurturing, supportive, and bonding principles at the center of things, where we stand, ruling the here and now.

These elemental forces interact with one another according to laws that are universal, and therefore predictable to some extent. The first three chapters and Chapter 7 of this book describe these laws of interaction with emphasis on the psychological level.

Third, we need to *train practitioners,* who are continually exposed to these types of energies, how to avoid being negatively affected by the by-products of treatments.[6]

There is no denying the fact that being constantly exposed to negative emotions is extremely draining. Anyone exposed to public work can testify to this. We don't even need to address the negativity in someone else, or even need to touch that person, to experience the negative effects. Sometimes just being in the mere presence of someone with a particular mindset can drain our vital energy and exhaust us. Whether we are massage therapists or psychotherapists, social workers or customer service clerks, schoolteachers or lawyers, if we come in contact with an unhappy public, we feel the need to "clean up" or "clear out" our own internal energy at the end of the day. The ancient Taoists discovered ways of transforming these energies, and recycling their negativity into positive life force. By extending these energies from internal life to the external environment, they gave us Feng-Shui, the Taoist esoteric art of landscaping, home arrangement, sacred architecture, and geomancy. By applying these energies to the body, they developed Kung-Fu, Nei-Kung, and Chi-Kung, the skills of mastering or managing our internal life. "Internal alchemy" (Nei-Dan), or the balancing of these elemental forces through our internal organs, gave birth to acupuncture and Chi Nei Tsang, the art of internal healing, or internally applied Chi-Kung.

Healing, Education, Depression, and Academia

Learning is a biological fact. It takes time for our nervous system to grow and establish good connections between neurons for new information to be integrated into the previous pattern of knowledge. The learning curve is exactly the same as the healing curve—it is an upward stairway curve (see Figure 3). It feels as though we have reached a plateau, or that we are even getting worse before we feel sudden improvement. We might feel confused, as if we no longer know anything, before we can eventually perform better than ever. For example, when we learn to play a piece of music, or to dance, when we learn a martial art technique, or a new computer program, first we fumble with it very poorly and then one day, the music comes out right, the dance or martial movement becomes smooth, and we don't need as much concentration to use the computer program. We work for a long time without feeling any progress, and then, all of a sudden, it comes. We don't really know why or what happened that caused this, but we don't question it, we just move on. This means that our nervous system has solidly integrated the new information.

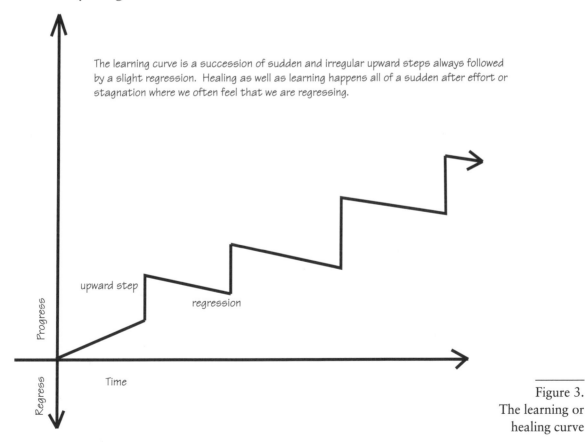

The learning curve is a succession of sudden and irregular upward steps always followed by a slight regression. Healing as well as learning happens all of a sudden after effort or stagnation where we often feel that we are regressing.

upward step

regression

Progress

Regress

Time

Figure 3.
The learning or
healing curve

The same holds true for healing. Most of us who subscribe to holistic healing modalities don't feel any improvement until we are actually at least 80 percent better. Only when we remember that the discomfort we used to feel all the time is now only occasional, do we realize that something is working. Because it is normal to feel good, when we get better we just feel normal.

All successful educators will tell you the same thing about learning: The only way to learn is by making mistakes. This is why playing while learning is so important. If we make mistakes as we play, it is not that important; there are no major consequences, and we can even make fun of our mistakes. This is the way a child learns naturally. A child is in a constant learning mode. If he doesn't learn, it is generally because of the teaching technique, or a negative emotional reaction to the educator, or a deficiency in the educational system as a whole. A certain amount of lightheartedness and enjoyment is essential for balance in the learning process. As soon as we are asked to be serious, we find it very difficult to learn. For example, the act of frowning closes our Microcosmic Orbit (see Chapter 5), the general receiving pathways of our meridian system, and makes it difficult, often impossible, to take in energy and information (Chi), or to be sympathetic. For this reason, it is used in combat: Frowning prevents soldiers from caring about what others feel. If you keep a frown on your face long enough, soon you won't be able to feel what's going on around you at all. Your feelings will automatically be transformed into thoughts by switching from a feeling state (Metal) to an analytical state (Wood). In this way, so-called frowning intellectuals (Wood) adopt the proud martial attitude and vocabulary of the warrior, becoming disconnected from the world of feelings and emotions (Metal). From this perspective, the more we think, the less we feel. The net result is a disassociation of the nonrational, abstract side of the self that makes up our emotional side, with the tendency to invalidate feelings.

As I stated earlier, we are not responsible for having emotions. We don't choose them; we get them. To have emotions or feelings invalidated is tantamount to being imprisoned. To the emotional self, not to have the right to feel means not to have the right to live. This is where depression comes into the picture.

I believe that depression is a chronic condition of our academic world. It is a legacy of the Renaissance period, the cultural attempt of Western civilization to step out of the dark ages of medieval times. The Western world, plagued with enormous suffering, found the escape offered by intellectualism, under the economic protection and privileged status of the royal courts of Europe, quite understandably irresistible. It was the birth of science, the preponderance of "I think, therefore I am," which has set the philosophical perspective of the academic sciences since the time of Déscartes.

We have inherited a culture that is chronically depressed and martially oriented, chronically intellectual and emotionally abusive. The mental attitude of seriousness without the balancing nature of playfulness, high spirit, and satisfaction prevents the learning process from unfolding in a healthy manner, making it extremely difficult for any educational system to work (see Chapter 7). Intellectuals will know a great deal from learning "by heart," and will be able to remember a tremendous amount of information. Because they are not able to feel completely satisfied outside of "intellectual satisfaction," however, they will be idealists and perfectionists, and they will have great difficulty proving emotional maturity using their knowledge. They will be great but impractical thinkers; great but emotionally irresponsible inventors; great but uncaring, unfeeling strategists with no sense of a true notion of respect, authenticity, or authority from experience and true knowledge called wisdom.

Emotional ignorance then sets in. Ignorant people are ignorant of ignorance; therefore, they don't know how much more they would know, and how much better they would feel without the affliction of ignorance. Even worse, being ignorant of ignorance makes ignorant people believe that they know everything! Ignorance is the source of arrogance. For the ignorant, no intellectual, logical, rational approach will be able to prove them wrong. So, what's the solution?

There is no solution because if we come from feeling instead of thinking, it is an emotional rather than an intellectual issue. It is then not rational, and therefore not solvable. It is not something that can just be explained away or solved by thinking; it is something that needs to be outgrown. That growth is a healing process that involves awareness, which is manifested as physical pain when it comes from a physical symptom, or as emotional-behavioral upset at the mental level. This is the healing crisis or the price of awareness in the first stage, awareness; confusion in the second stage, resetting the mind; transformation in the third stage, change; and surrender in the fourth stage, acceptance of change. Without completion of these four distinct stages, no healing is possible (see Chapter 8), only a permanent state of emotional immaturity, insensitivity, and depression.

Earth Relationship Chi-Kung

This is the first exercise I always teach students. It involves bringing awareness of the way we are made to feel about the earth and its attributes of solidity, consistency, balance, harmony, nurturing, and the ability to be comfortable in the present, to be able to feel at the right place, at the right time, and doing the right thing with the right people.

Mentally, we might feel good about the idea, but witnessing how our physical body reacts during the exercise and the difficulty we might experience in following the instructions will put us in touch with the unconscious way we feel about the relationship we really have with the elemental entity of earth.

1. Calmly and rhythmically shake your body, becoming aware of your bones differentiated from your muscles. Sink as you inhale, and push your feet into the ground as you exhale and rise. Be aware of how strange and unnatural this feels. The natural tendency in our modern culture—I no longer call it Western because this tendency has spread to much of the rest of the world—is to do the reverse: to lift off during inhale and stay afloat as long as possible during exhale with the net result of losing the feeling of connection with the earth.

2. Keep shaking and sinking as you inhale and keep pushing your feet into the ground as you exhale, as if you want to leave deep footprints in the ground. Do it intentionally and energetically for a few times until it becomes automatic. Then let your body relax, and witness how, as you exhale, you can relax more of your body weight into the ground. Try to get rid of tensions you don't need in order to remain standing.

3. As you keep shaking and sinking your body weight as you inhale and pushing your body weight into the ground as you exhale,

be aware of the "pushing back" from the ground. This pushing back is actually the resistance to your push and represents how solidly the earth supports you. Take that feeling of support deep within you and relax more of your body into it. Be aware of the unconditional nature of this support and relax into it completely. Feel it in your feet and relax them completely. Feel the earth support inside your legs and pelvis, in the whole length of your spine, and even in your ribs, your sternum, your shoulders, your jaws, and your neck. Progressively, let the entire weight of your body sink into that unconditional support from the earth.

4. Smile in your feet. Soften your feet and smile there. Smiling is contagious. Soon you will experience the softening of the ground under your feet. This is the earth smiling back at you. Take that softness deep within you.

Be aware of the difficulty of the exercise. Even if you are not able to let go of all tensions related to holding yourself up instead of letting the earth hold you, tell yourself that from now on, you will experiment at getting better every day a little bit at a time. It is normal not to be able to relax our weight into the earth. We were made not to trust the support of the earth. Earth is often unstable and slippery, and when we fall, it hurts! Earth is dirty; there are germs and bugs there. And it is hard and uncomfortable. We don't want to smell it, much less taste it. There is even something morally wrong about the idea of tasting the earth! It is nothing rational even though we can easily justify it. It is just the way we feel about it, and there is nothing wrong with that. The only thing wrong is not to be aware of it! The difference between animals, like a dog for example, and us, is that the dog, when tired, will stop anywhere more or less hospitable and turn around several times before lying down and falling asleep immediately. The dog adapts itself to the conditions of the earth. We humans, on the other hand, will first have to flatten the place, and then put down several layers of padding to make the earth comfortable for us. We adapt the earth to our need to feel comfortable. Again, there is nothing wrong with that. The only thing is that when we don't know how uncomfortable we really feel with ourselves, it won't matter how much we adapt or change the earth, or how much padding we put down. We will never feel comfortable enough or satisfied, no matter what. This is how we end up becoming abusive with our environment!

Similarly, in our own bodies, we learn to compensate by holding ourselves instead of letting the earth hold us. The more we have to hold ourselves, the less we trust the earth for support. The less we trust the earth for support, the less we trust anything or anyone else for support. Not the ground, not our parents, not our friends, not any authority figures, even though somewhere deep inside we long for it. This is what we carry in the shadow of our psyche when we are unaware of what we do. Not being able to relax and trust the earth for support translates, in our emotional self, into not trusting anything, including the earth within us, the way we feel about ourselves. This has a far-reaching influence on our self-esteem and the way we interact with others.

By doing this simple Earth Relationship Chi-Kung every day, you will begin to trust the earth more. This will transform the way you stand up for yourself, it will give you a clear perspective on life, and help you develop a sense of ease and comfort both in your habitat and in your relationships. Practicing this meditation regularly will make you feel at home in any kind of situation.

Chapter ★ 2

Taoist Cosmology and the Five Elemental Forces of Existence

Cosmology

Color plates 1, 2, 3, 4, and 5 illustrate the points made in this chapter. The color plates are printed together in the center of this book.

Wu-Chi

Thousands of years ago, the ancient Taoists described this universe as ever expanding and cyclical, long before modern Western physicists posited the Big Bang theory. Our Chinese forefathers in Taoist studies and Chi-Kung already had a very accurate awareness of how our universe came into existence, even though their experience stemmed more from the introspective study of the inner universe through the I'Ching than from exploring the outer universe with telescopes and mathematics. In fact, they were already in touch with abstract concepts, which we in the modern West only started to comprehend very recently through the theories of relativity and quantum physics. The study of the I'Ching becomes even more relevant today with a better understanding of genetics and DNA.[7]

Before anything existed, there was *nothing,* called *Wu-Chi* in Chinese. That nothingness is absolute so we can't even say that it came before time, since neither time nor space exists in Wu-Chi. Out of this nothingness comes *Tai-Chi,* our universe of space and time, our universe of dimensions, duration of past, present, and future, planets and galaxies, the birth of history and existence that came within moments of the Big Bang, which gave birth to our still expanding universe.

The theory of relativity states that if right now we were riding that ever-expanding wave of creation at the limit of our universe and looking at its center, we would be witnessing its birth, the Big Bang itself. We would still be experiencing the beginning of time. "Beyond" is Wu-Chi, and, at the center, at its origin, is also Wu-Chi. We can say then that Wu-Chi is the origin of our universe and, at the same time, that Wu-Chi also "contains" it. Wu-Chi can't be localized physically since our laws of physics don't apply to it. It is nowhere and everywhere at the same time. It can only be mathematically perceived like the center of a wheel in motion that requires a perfectly still center for its very existence, but is invisible to the naked eye and nowhere to be found at the strictly physical level.

Being the absolute origin, Wu-Chi "contains" all the information and energy of the universe required for its existence, and is also at the "center" of everything. Wu-Chi is then a nontemporal, nonlocal, absolute source of energy and information: the definition of God, the creator of existence. Strictly speaking from a Taoist perspective, existence comes out of "no-where" to "now-here," here and now, and consistently returns to it, from Absolute Spirit to the universe of dimensions and back again.

Tai-Chi

Tai-Chi is our universe, the universe of dualities, polarities, distance, time, and space. It is the cosmos with its ever-expanding edge, and its stars, planets, and galaxies. It is the universe of planet Earth and its ecosystems. It is the universe of humanity, its history, evolution, tribulations, and revolutions. It is also the kosmos, for lack of a better word. *Kosmos,* as opposed to *cosmos,* refers to the deepest stratum of the internal universe as well as the full external range of the outer universe. The *kosmic* aspect of existence covers not only the microcosmic and macrocosmic aspects of the material universe, but also the not-so-obvious, yet nevertheless very important aspects of the spiritual world, including the informational universe contained in our genetic background.

Tai-Chi is a cyclical universe, powered by Chi, and ever alternating from Yin to Yang and from Yang to Yin. As a current of electricity is inseparable from the polarities that create it, Chi is inseparable from the continuous cycle of Yin and Yang. Within extreme Yang, we always find Yin, and within extreme Yin, we always find Yang. It is the cycle of history, the cycle of years, the cycle of life and death—very rhythmic, very constant. Laws of existence rule this universe. They are the laws of physics, the forces of nature, and all the laws known by the ancient Taoists as the universal truth or, to paraphrase Master Ni, the "Unchanging Law of Changes."[8] These are laws of attraction, repulsion, opposition, and indifference—everything that composes the manifestations of life, and the studies of which constitute the I'Ching.

The universe of Tai-Chi is composed of the Five Elemental Forces of Nature that create the alchemy of life. These elemental forces are responsible for life and its manifestations. They are composed of the basic elements of Tai-Chi, our universe: Water for extreme Yin, what is essential, deep, hidden, cold, and dark; and Fire for extreme Yang, what is consistent, superficial, apparent, hot, and bright. These are the two basic phases of Tai-Chi from Yin-cold to Yang-hot. To get from Yin-cold to Yang-hot, we have a warming-up, expanding phase called Wood, and to get from Yang-hot to Yin-cold, we have a cooling-down, constrictive phase called Metal. Earth is the central place of observation, the ever-present moment, the immutable center of the turning wheel.

Tai-Chi also represents the cycles of the year, the seasons and the cardinal directions with the summer solstice at the extreme Yang (Fire) and the southern direction, the winter solstice at the extreme Yin (Water) and the northern direction, the spring equinox at the eastern direction of the rising sun (Wood), and the fall equinox at the western direction of the setting sun (Metal). A period of one year, the time the planet Earth takes to make a complete revolution around the sun, consists of thirteen months, the time it takes the moon to revolve around the Earth while the Earth revolves around the sun. Each month consists of twenty-eight days or four quarters of moon (weeks). Each season is three months. The thirteenth month is the week of transition between the seasons. This is the Earth season, the time for adaptation and balance. The Earth season is predominantly felt during that time in between summer and fall we call the harvest season, or Indian summer—the season of abundance, comfort, and calm between the heat of summer and the chill and rains of fall. Remember, however, that the

Earth season also exists between the seasons. It is the center, the place of observation, the here and now—not in the past, nor in the future, but in the eternity of the present moment.

The Five Elemental Forces of Nature, of Existence, of Life

Out of Tai-Chi comes life. Life is what happens when the Five Elemental Forces of Nature work together in harmony.

- From Water, we get our genetic background, reproduction, instinct, willpower, vision, and dreams.
- From Wood, we get our intelligence and potential for growth and cultivation.
- From Fire, we get our spirit, guidance, consciousness, intuition, and wisdom.
- From Earth, we get authenticity, our ability to be solid and comfortable in the present so that we are clever, spontaneous, practical, and adaptable.
- From Metal, we get our valor and pride, and our sensitivity to emotions so that our soul can grow from our life experience.

The 10,000 Things, or the Manifestations of Life

Once we have life, then come the manifestations of life and the interconnectedness with everything that constitutes existence. For our Taoist ancestors, life was more broadly defined than in our modern Western, conventionally accepted idea of life. According to the Taoists, every ecosystem, every part of every ecosystem, has a life of its own. The life of a wild animal, such as a deer or a bird, is dependent on the life of the entire forest it lives in. The forest is dependent on the life of the mountain where that forest grows. Thus, from the ancient Taoist perspective, forest and mountain are both considered "alive," with a soul and spirit. Our individual lives cannot be conceived without the proper harmony of our metabolism. Similarly, from a Taoist perspective, every single part of our body is human and reflects our personality, and the life of the community to which we belong reflects the soul and spirit of that community and has to be harmonious and complete to support our health.

The Essence of Life and the Elemental Force of Water

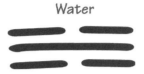

Water

Figure 4.
Water trigram

Water is our life force, the water of life. Water is the essence of life and death within us. When we die healthy, we die from kidney failure (our Yin Water organ); we have reached the end of our life potential as predetermined by our genes (Jing, stored in Kidneys, according to Traditional Chinese Medicine). Our kidneys just quit their basic function of maintaining our blood's pH balance, and we die painlessly and peacefully.

In an attempt to attain longevity, we try to strengthen our Water power with herbs and special exercises. Too much energy, however, can be very dangerous. Our system closely monitors the amount of energy we have available according to our lifestyle. Too much energy can kill us faster than too little. If we raise our energy with Chi-Kung or by taking a lot of ginseng, we want to make sure that we spend that energy. Practicing just for the sake of building energy can be extremely dangerous. Too much energy can bottleneck in zones of tension, creating a lot of pressure while giving us the feeling that energy is low because it is not circulating, as is the case with chronic fatigue syndrome. Then, when we take more ginseng, we don't feel any better and often develop worse symptoms. If we are otherwise healthy, when we are tired because of stagnant energy, increasing energy with herbs can bring the pressure to a breaking point and can put us at risk of a heart attack or a stroke. It is much better to assist the circulation of Chi by reducing its flow, and even stopping it at intervals to give it a rhythm, the same way a traffic light momentarily stops the flow of traffic to ease congestion. People with chronic fatigue have to learn to weave long periods of rest between all activities. They have to arrange the rhythm of their daily life around their meals and resting time the way healthy people normally do. In Taoist alchemical terms, it is letting our inner Earth control our inner Water.

Water is the force of creation, the power of originality, creativity, effortless progress. When our Water Chi is abundant, new ideas come easily to us, and we trust our instinct; we feel very strong, and very powerful. Out of this sense of power come calm and gentleness. But if our Water is scarce, then we can't help but be afraid. We'll have a deep feeling of weakness, which will automatically make us afraid of anything. Once we are afraid, it is easy to find reasons to be even more afraid. We'll also feel chronically needy and often frantic about getting what we want. From this come aggressiveness, entitlement issues, envy, jealousy, vindictiveness, paranoia, abuse, and violence.

The Water Principle

Water represents the extreme Yin part of Tai-Chi and is the most essential condition for life. All the research conducted by NASA to find signs of potential life elsewhere in the universe has been directed primarily at searching for water on other planets.

Water is represented in the I'Ching by "extreme Yin": Yang within Yin, the smallest Yang influence possible. Water runs deep, sinks naturally without being forced, is cold, hidden, fluid, and soft. It is the dormant seed in the winter, which contains all the life force of the mighty tree to come. It is extremely gentle, but all-powerful; nothing can resist its constant push or its yearning to spring forth. It contains the power of the tidal wave, which surges continually without retracting. It is the power of creation itself, the forces of sensuality, of life-giving force, of creativity, and willpower.

Water is manifested in the northern direction and the winter season.

In the body, Water is the most essential element of life: it holds our DNA, a generic term for our genes. It contains our genetic background (prenatal Chi), and is responsible for our potential for life. In Traditional Chinese Medicine, it is called Kidneys, or more accurately, our Yin Water Function, and circulates with the help of its Yang-associated organ, the Urinary Bladder, our Yang Water Function. Water affects the health of our kidneys, our bones, our marrow and brain, our urinary and reproductive systems, and our ability to hear and listen. Water also affects our ability to have instinct, dreams, hope, foresight, and determination.

When our Water Chi is healthy and plentiful, we have a solid genetic background, a rich cultural heritage. When we benefit from a solid support system (Earth supports and directs Water) from our parents, from friends and peers, from our community and government, life comes easily to us, and we feel calm, without the need to fight. Our will is strong and our behavior is gentle. We are already born winners.

When our Water Chi is poor, we are in survival mode. Our entire system is ready for "fight or flight." We feel so weak that even when we are ready to fight, we know that we are going to lose. Flooded with adrenaline and stress hormones, we live in fear, and we are prone to fits of despair, anger, or depression, easily feeling discouraged and powerless.

Water nourishes Wood, controls Fire, and can only be efficiently contained by Earth.

In Water, we find our dreams.

Mental aspects: instinct, creativity.

Positive emotional qualities and feelings: gentle, soft, prudent, limitless, encompassing, embracing, calm, determined, creative, sensual.

Negative emotional qualities and feelings: impulsive, fearful, cold, rough, slippery, small, scattered, timid, absent, speedy, stagnant, running in circles, sterile, lewd, paranoid.

Water symptoms: dark circles around the eyes, weakness in the legs, lower back pain, fatigue, bad teeth, weak knees, loss of hearing, frequent urination, osteoporosis, kidney stones.

Power animals: Since we have two kidneys, we also have two power animals for Water: the water turtle and the deer (or goat in mountain cultures). The turtle represents longevity, endurance, and genetic strength; the deer represents sexual vigor and vitality.

Arts: painting, drawing and sculpture, figurative arts in general, photography and film, the arts that bring the essence of life to figures and manifest the power of abstraction and dreams.

Occupations: All work related to finance, banking, accounting, investment, retail, and real estate. Also, professions related to travel and tourism.

Language: symbols.

Water Meditation

The best way to do any kind of elemental force meditation is to be right in front of or near a manifestation of that element to allow all of your senses to make direct contact. Nevertheless, imagination and visualization can also be very strong. However, never miss an opportunity to be near a real waterfall, a beautiful lake, or by the ocean.

For each element, we are going to first use the *inner smile* to help relax and trigger the parasympathetic response, the healing response of the body. Smiling is very powerful: anywhere you can smile inside yourself makes that part more relaxed and more alkaline. It is much more effective and immediate than any kind of special diet to make your blood more alkaline. The stress response itself is acidic because neurotransmitters and stress hormones are acidic. The inner smile has the power to instantly reverse the effects of the stress response in our body. It just has to be done with heart, authenticity, and consistency. To the inner smile, we add a color specific to that elemental force and run it through the bodily systems related to that element to enhance their health.

- Sit or stand comfortably. Bring your mind to your center; close your eyes and be aware of your mid-eyebrow. Relax your mid-eyebrow, relax your whole forehead, and let a smile come to your face. Relax your eyes, your forehead, your lips, your jaws, and slightly raise the corners of your mouth. Picture a smile right on your mid-eyebrow. It can be a very familiar smile of someone you love, or a smile seen recently, a very authentic smile, like a young child's or baby's smile—very genuine, very clear, very distinct. Picture there also, on your mid-eyebrow, a deep blue light, very deep and very blue like the deep ocean or a deep lake.

- So, now you see that deep blue light with a big smile on it right on your mid-eyebrow. Slowly, bring the deep blue light and the smile to your ears, inside your ears. Let them sink deep into your ears so you feel the smile and the deep blue light filling up your ears and slowly sinking very deep inside, so deep that you reach inwardly all the way down to your kidneys. There is a direct connection there between your ears and your kidneys, very easy to find.

- Feel your kidneys relaxing and filling up with that big smile and the deep blue light. Feel and maintain that connection between your ears and your kidneys.

- Feel the smile and the deep blue light flowing from your ears to your kidneys and down to your lower abdomen, all the way to your bladder on your pelvic floor, your sexual organs, and your reproductive organs where it builds like a deep pool of deep blue water with a big smile in it.

- Feel the coolness all the way from your ears down to your kidneys, down to your lower abdomen, and bring the same feeling inside your bones.

- Feel all your bones filled up with cool deep blue water. Feel the coolness, feel the weight. Smile in your bones. So, now you feel the smile and the deep blue light from your ears to your kidneys, down to your lower abdomen, and inside all your bones.

- Be aware of the power of Water, very strong but extremely gentle, the power of gentleness. It's the power of sinking, following the path of least resistance, and springing forth effortlessly. It's the power of life-giving force, the power of creativity, of will. It's the power of Yang within Yin, which emerges in the power of the surge of sap in trees in the spring, the power of the wave, the surf.

- Feel that power in your kidneys and your ears, feel it in your lower abdomen and your bones. Feel the power of the whole ocean inside your kidneys.

- Bring in front of you your ideal representation of Water, the archetype of Water, with its sounds, smell, movement, sensation. It can be the ocean, a wave of the ocean, a lake, a river or stream, a waterfall, rain—the universal power of Water.

- Pull the universal power of Water inside your own water system in your body, feeling its manifestation inside your kidneys, your ears, your genitals, your whole lower abdomen and perineum, and in all your bones.

- Keep the work of this meditation deep within you.

The Power of Cultivation and the Elemental Force of Wood

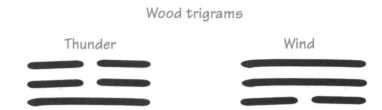

Wood trigrams

Thunder   Wind

Figure 5.
Thunder and
Wind trigrams

Wood is our intelligence. Once we conceive ideas with Water, then we can develop them into theories, plans, and strategies with Wood. Wood is everything that grows, that can be ameliorated or cultivated. It carries the power of the mind, the thinking mind, the power of intelligence and clarity. In our body, it is our nervous system. Even though we lose neurons every day, even though we age, even though we stop growing, our nervous system continues to grow connections. Old remaining neurons continue growing new dendrites and making new synapses inside our body. This is the reason old masters—master potters, dancers, martial artists, musicians—are always the best at what they do. It is because they have been doing it longer than anyone else. If we compare masters with their students, or older and more experienced artists with younger, less experienced ones, we find that anything involving real art, refinement, and dexterity will be carried out with the ease of a master rather than with the effort of a student.

Wood can only grow and grow, like our ability to think, to analyze, to clarify, to ameliorate. Wood is the very reason why perfection itself doesn't exist in this universe of Tai-Chi because everything can be and does get perfected; everything can evolve and grow without end.

Wood is abundance and generosity. The symbol for Wood is the tree. In order to reproduce, the tree needs only one seed. Look at all the seeds of one tree and all the blossoms and the fruit. Look at how the tree provides shelter and food for birds, butterflies, and other animals; it even provides protective and cooling shade. A tree is, in itself, an entire ecosystem.

The Wood Principle

Wood represents the complete warming-up phase from extreme Yin-cold to extreme Yang-hot, from Water to Fire. It is everything that grows, expands, enriches, warms, and multiplies. It is the full phase of growth from seed (Water) to blossom (Fire). From roots to sprouts and stem, to branches and leaves—all are Wood. It is generosity itself, the spirit of youth, of fecundity, reproduction, and sexual drive.

Wood is manifested in the eastern direction (the rising sun) and the spring season.

In the body, it is first and foremost our nervous system, the only system that can't stop working and growing without sustaining permanent damage. Compared to other systems in our body, if our nervous system stops growing, we lose it. On the other hand, repetitive and constant activity is the worst thing for our nervous system. If we feel nervously tired because of working too long on a project, the best way to rest is *not* to lie down and do nothing. If we do this, our mind will start obsessing about the project and, because its "fuel supply" has been cut off, it will be unable to further evolve and conceive new ideas. Therefore, the best way to rest our nervous system is to ease into relaxation by changing activities. We should play or listen to music, read a novel, play a game, daydream—do anything that will keep our mind busy with something else, and the mind will rest more efficiently than if we try to stop thinking altogether.

Wood is the power of thinking: observation, research, vigilance, and clarifying. And Wood is the power of intelligence: problem solving, planning, strategizing, analyzing, and composing. Its power resides in the Liver, our Yin Wood organ, and it is circulated by the Gallbladder, our Yang Wood organ. Wood affects the health of our liver, especially its ability to deal with toxicity, as well as our nerves, our sex drive, our ability to think clearly, and our eyesight.

When our Wood Chi is healthy and abundant, we have clarity of mind and a high power of focus. The mental strength fed by creativity (Water feeds Wood) allows us to cover the full spectrum of possibilities, theories, and strategies, and our capacity for problem solving is acute and precise.

When our Wood Chi is unhealthy or deficient, we lose perspective and become confused. We often become victim of delusion with mental focus turning into obsession. This can then lead to impulsiveness, aggressiveness, and fits of anger.

Wood feeds Fire, controls Earth, and is controlled by Metal.

In Wood, we find our mental self.

Mental aspects: thinking, intelligence, rationality, focused attention, strategy, planning, and management.

Positive emotional qualities and feelings: clear-minded, generous, kind, tempered, intelligent, cool-headed, pleasant, humble, discreet, relaxed, progressive, constructive, cooperative, conciliatory, open-minded.

Negative emotional qualities and feelings: obscure, vindictive, aggressive, stingy, violent, strategic, hot-headed, explosive, tight, obstreperous, obsessed, obstinate, formalistic, dogmatic, arrogant, utopian, competitive, antagonistic, narrow-minded.

Wood symptoms: intoxication, addictions, allergies, bad digestion, bad breath coming from bad digestion, pimples, yellowish or greenish hue of the skin.

Power animal: In old Taoist Chinese tradition, the mythical dragon holds the Wood power. The dragon in Eastern tradition is much different than the scary Western dragon. The Western dragon plunders and hoards riches in a deep mountain cave, and is reminiscent of our fascination with monsters and dinosaurs, which are more representative of the dark side of our psyche. The Asian dragon is a happy dragon. It brings good luck and prosperity. During Chinese New Year celebrations, it is a common sight to see the Asian dragon winding its way through the streets of Chinatowns, and to see its face displayed as a mask in most businesses. The dragon is a mythical animal with the body of the sensuous fish, the head of the intelligent and disciplined horse, the whiskers of the great-hearted lion, the claws of the forceful eagle, and the tail of the luscious snake. The dragon does indeed carry all the attributes and qualities of these different animals.

Arts: poetry and writing, and, of course, martial arts, athletics, and sports in general.

Occupations: All work related to management, politics, lobbying, critiquing, military, law enforcement, and the judicial system.

Language: pictures, images.

Wood Meditation

- Sit or stand comfortably. Bring your mind to your center, close your eyes, and be aware of your mid-eyebrow. Relax your mid-eyebrow, relax your whole forehead, and let a smile come to your face. Relax your eyes, lips, and jaws, and slightly raise the corners of your mouth. Picture a smile right on your mid-eyebrow. It can be a very familiar smile of someone you love, or a smile seen recently, a very authentic smile, like a young child's or baby's smile—very genuine, very clear, very distinct. Picture there also, on your mid-eyebrow, a very bright green light, very bright and very green like the sun shining on a tropical rain forest right after the rain—very vibrant, very green, very lush.

- So, now you can see a bright green light on your mid-eyebrow, with a big smile on it. From your mid-eyebrow, spread the bright green light and the smile to your eyes and draw them in and feel the greenness, feel the lushness filling up your eyes with a green light that is both calming and invigorating, like the luminous green of a wheat field in the spring sun, and a smile all the way back to your optic nerves.

- Feel the bright green light and the big smile spreading from your eyes to your optic nerves and filling up your brain. Feel your brain relaxing, feel the soothing green light shining inside your whole brain and then down your spinal cord to all the nerves in your body; all the way to the surface of your skin, to each nerve plexus, to all your organs. Feel all your nerves relaxing and turning bright green and smiling.

- Look inward at your liver and gallbladder, and smile at them. Keep smiling until they smile back at you. Smiling is contagious. Give a sincere and authentic smile to your liver, and it will smile back at you. Flash the bright green light throughout the whole volume of your liver and gallbladder. If you find any dark spots there, keep flashing the bright green light on them.

- Be aware of the power of Wood: the power of cultivation, the power of understanding, the power of thoughts and clarity of mind, the power to always understand better and more clearly. It is a very generous power: the power to grow enough so that you can give and share. It is the power of kindness and generosity. Feel it in your eyes, brain, spinal cord, and all your nerves. Feel it in your liver and gallbladder.

- In front of you, you are going to picture your ideal representation of Wood. It could be your favorite tree, an archetype of trees, a whole forest, or it could be your favorite plant. Picture it very healthy, very lush with thick foliage and blossoms and fruit. Be aware of the greenness and brightness of the foliage.

- Draw its power inside your own Wood system, inside your eyes, throughout all your nerves, bathing your brain in it. Feel your whole liver filling up with that power.

- Feel your Wood power regenerated. Feel your nervous system cleaned up, your thinking calm and clear.

- Keep the work of this meditation deep within you.

Guidance and High Spirit and the Elemental Force of Fire

Fire

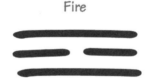

Figure 6.
Fire trigram

Chi grows from extreme Yin in Water to extreme Yang in Fire, passing through all the different phases of growth and warming up in Wood. Fire is the blooming phase. The spiritual insight comes from the wisdom acquired through intellectual development in Wood.

The Fire Principle

Fire represents the extreme Yang part of the universe (Tai-Chi). It is represented in the I'Ching by Yin within Yang, the smallest Yin influence possible. There is no absolute in this universe of Tai-Chi. Fire is bright and hot, obvious and consistent, substantial and loud, explosive and burning. It is the phase of blossom and attainment, with its brightness and radiance overpowering.

Fire is manifested in the southern direction and the summer season.

In the body, it is what we give the most importance to: the heart. It contains our spirit and is responsible for our enjoyment of life. In

Traditional Chinese Medicine, Fire manifests itself in two different systems: the cardiovascular system with the Heart, our Yin Fire organ, and the Small Intestine, our Yang Fire organ, where it is circulated; and the endocrine system with the Heart Controller, our Yin Fire organ (also called Pericardium, Heart Constrictor, and Circulation Sex), which is circulated through our Triple Burner or Triple Heater, our Yang Fire organ, responsible for harmonizing the three main phases of our Chi: distribution of Chi (first burner), extraction of Chi (second burner), and elimination/storage/transformation of Chi (third burner). Fire affects the health of our cardiovascular system, our blood, our endocrine system, and our ability to communicate within and without. It is responsible for the brightness of our spirit and holds the torch that guides us on the path of our life purpose.

When our inner Fire is healthy and bright, we have high spirit. Our intuition and enthusiasm for life always guide us to the right place at the right time to meet the right people (Fire controls Earth). We feel joy and a strong sense of purpose in our life.

When our Fire Chi is perturbed or weak, we lose faith in ourselves, in others, and in life in general. We lack enthusiasm and direction in life. Unable to reach out and connect with others, or communicate our inner feelings, we are helpless and unable to help anyone else. We lose touch and sensitivity (Fire controls Metal); we become emotionless, and often uncaring and cruel.

Fire nurtures Earth, tempers Metal, and is controlled by Water.

In Fire, we find our spirit.

Mental aspects: communication, intuition, consciousness, and guidance.

Positive emotional qualities and feelings: compassionate, joyful, spiritual, hearty, passionate, enthusiastic, respectful, polite, refined, patient, bright, loving, forgiving.

Negative emotional qualities and feelings: impatient, hasty, insensitive, cynical, hateful, spiteful, cruel, vicious, inconsiderate, mocking, thoughtless, tasteless, obsessed, obsequious.

Fire symptoms: high or low blood pressure, pain in the chest or in the back behind the heart, buzzing in the ears, bloodshot eyes, red or white nose, shortness of breath, flushed complexion, hastiness, always hurrying.

Power animal: The ancient Taoist mythical animal associated with Fire is the phoenix. However, I find the attributes of Fire in many birds like the hummingbird, and often other red-throated birds, which dance, sing, and fly very high merely for the sake of enjoying themselves. The eagle and the mythical thunderbird are also connected with spiritual Fire.

Arts: dance, song, mime, acting, theatre, opera, drama, comedy, performing arts in general.

Occupations: All work connected with leadership, masters, teachers, spiritual leaders, and priests. Also all work related to medicine, healing, birthing and child-rearing, and education. And all work related to the performing arts, show business, and entertainment.

Language: A very short vocabulary. The language of intuition, and of extremes, which typically is expressed extremely simply—yes or no, like or dislike, go or don't go.

Awaken Your Inner Fire Meditation

This meditation is to enhance the power of your heart. It reverses depression, increases vitality, gives enthusiasm for life, and rekindles passion. If you are impatient, it also helps to soften your heart so that you can enjoy the present moment more fully. When practiced regularly, this meditation will have the same effect as an acupuncture treatment for your heart and will protect your whole cardiovascular system from imbalance and disease.

- Find a comfortable sitting position with your back straight but not stiff. Center your breath and your mind behind your navel and breathe fully but slowly.

- Feel the support of the earth beneath you. Let the weight of your body sink as you inhale and push your weight comfortably down into the earth as you exhale. Feel the pushing back of that support from the earth and take in that feeling of unconditional support deep within you.

- Bring your mind to your center; close your eyes and be aware of your mid-eyebrow. Relax your mid-eyebrow, relax your whole forehead, and let a smile come to your face. Relax your eyes, your lips, your jaws, and slightly raise the corners of your mouth. Picture a smile right on your mid-eyebrow. It can be a very familiar smile of someone you love, or a smile seen recently, a very authentic smile like a young child's or baby's smile—very genuine, very clear, very distinct.

- Between your eyes, picture a big smile and a bright red light— very bright, very red, like the tropical sun shining on a bright red hibiscus flower.

- Take the time to observe that bright red light with the big smile on it. Make it very real, very clear, very distinct.

- Bring that bright red light and the smile to your tongue and let it relax and swell up with the red light. Feel it very red, very warm. Feel the smile in it as if you were just about to say something very nice, or as if you were just about to sing your favorite song.

- Keep that nice feeling in your tongue and bring that big smile and the bright red light directly from your tongue to your heart. There is a direct connection there, very easy to find. Feel your heart swelling up with the big smile and the bright red light.

- Let the bright red light and the smile fill up your heart and expand to all the arteries, all the veins, all the blood vessels in your body. Feel the warmth in them, feel them relaxing as you smile through them.

- Bring the same feeling, the same warmth to your thymus, that gland above your heart in your chest that protects your health. Smile in it and send the bright red light there until you feel it swelling in your chest.

- Bring the same bright red light, the same big smile, and that same feeling of warmth to your small intestine, the shyest organ in your body, the dwelling place of your spirit, that inner guide that gives you gut feelings. Smile in it and embrace it in your body. Feel the warmth in it, and let that warmth spread up to your heart and to all your blood.

- Feel every single blood cell in your body smiling. Feel them very red and bright, very happy.

- Keep that pleasant feeling of warmth, the bright red light, and the smile in your blood, your small intestine, your thymus, your heart, and your tongue together.

- Next, be aware of the place in your back right behind your heart. This is your fourth thoracic vertebra. Feel this area; it is your center of freedom. Breathe and let go of any heaviness there. If you feel tense, or if you are not able to breathe and relax there, go deep within yourself and try to get a sense of what you do, or what is done to you, that burdens you there. Feel what you can do to start bringing a change there so that this part of your back can start loosening, freeing itself from whatever is restricting your feeling of freedom and liberty, whatever is holding back your spirit.

- Next, be aware of your tongue and your heart and feel the internal connection between them. Breathe and smile to that space. Feel your tongue directly connected to your heart. Make sure there is a tight connection there and let your tongue speak only the truth of your spirit. Make sure there is no obstruction that could prevent you from releasing any burden from your heart.

- In front of you, visualize a beautiful fire—very bright, warm, and majestic, the most beautiful fire you can imagine, the archetype of all fires. Make it very clear, very distinct, and right in front of you.

- Then go back within yourself and observe your personal Fire in your heart, in your blood, in your guts, in your tongue, and your heart together. Observe it carefully and be aware of places where it could be a little brighter, or warmer. Be aware of places where it doesn't feel so hot, where it feels a little weak.

- Feel the archetype of Fire in front of you and absorb its energy. Draw its warmth and its brightness directly into these places within your own Fire system that need it. Take your time and send the warmth and brightness to the most remote places at the bottom of your heart, in your veins and the depth of your gut, and revive the flames there.

- Feel all your inner Fire rekindled as if fueled with a richer octane, a fire that burns very clean, a fire that leaves no smoke. Feel it in all your blood cells, running through your veins; feel it in your gut, feel it in your heart and your tongue together.

- Between your eyebrows, bring back a big smile and also picture a bright purple light—very bright and very purple, like a beautiful purple star shining joyfully between your eyebrows. Make it so purple, so bright, and so intense that it can be seen all the way from outer space.

- Very slowly, very carefully, draw in the smile and the purple light to all the principle endocrine glands in your body corresponding to the major centers of information and energy. These places are called Chakras in the Eastern tradition.

- From your mid-eyebrow, draw the bright purple light and your smile to the very center of your head, at the base of your brain where your pineal and pituitary glands are, and make them shine like a star that can be seen from outer space.

- Also draw the bright purple light and the smile to your thyroid in your throat. Feel your whole throat relaxing, opening in all directions like a lotus in full bloom, radiating the purple light in all directions.

- Draw the inner smile and the purple light into your thymus in your chest. Feel any resistance there melting; feel the warmth, the smile and the purple light shining in all directions.

- Bring the purple light and the smile to your solar plexus, that complex region below your sternum, where your pancreas and liver connect to your duodenum, the crossroads to your feelings and emotions. Smile in there, drawing in the purple light until it shines brightly and clearly.

- Feel your adrenals above your kidneys. Smile at them and shine the purple light in them until they smile back at you and start shining and radiating the purple light on their own.

- Be aware of your reproductive glands in your lower abdomen— ovaries for women and testes for men. Feel them smiling, relaxing, shining a strong purple light.

- Be aware of all your main endocrine glands connected by the purple light and the inner smile, circulating together like a current from one to the other, from the top of your head to your pelvic floor, balancing the whole endocrine response, and harmonizing all the hormones. Feel them shining very brightly, like a purple constellation.

- Feel all the endocrine glands covering for one another. If one of the glands feels weak, even if one of them has been surgically removed, the added energy brought by this meditation will help compensate for the missing function. Feel the light burning more clearly and more brightly in these areas of weakness.

- Go deep within yourself and be aware of the power of Fire: the power of high spirit, the power of joy, of enthusiasm, of passion; the power of love, of caring; the power of warmth, of meaningful communication, of intuition, and consciousness. Feel it in your whole endocrine system: your pituitary, pineal, thyroid, thymus, pancreas, adrenals, and reproductive glands, and also in every endocrine function present in every organ, every tissue, every cell in your body. Feel the power of Fire in your blood, your gut, your heart, and your tongue together. Feel your inner Fire burning brightly and clearly.

- Feel the connection to the ground from your pelvic floor and feel the top of your head open. Send your best wishes and prayers from there. Send your questions, ask for help to solve a problem, ask for inspiration and guidance.

- Keep feeling your inner Fire burning cleanly. Feel the warmth of inner peace in your heart and the whole chain of Chakras.

- Keep the memory of this meditation deep within you.

The Power of Satisfaction and the Elemental Force of Earth

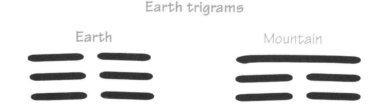

Earth trigrams

Earth   Mountain

Figure 7.
Earth and Mountain
trigrams

Following the burning phase of Fire, the Chi settles and ashes feed the earth with a revived potential for life. The wisdom of Fire becomes a sound common sense in Earth, allowing practical and harmonious manifestation and creations.

Earth is the principle of harmony, nurturing, support, and satisfaction. Earth is the place where we stand, the central place of absolute perspective, solidity, and unconditional support. It is the mid-point of balance and, for this reason, can be found in all places between stages and phases, and between seasons. Its influence is most prominent during harvest season, at the end of summer, when it is no longer too hot and not yet too cold, a time of plenty and comfort.

In our bodies, Earth is our flesh, our muscles, what we first associate with being our bodies. It is what we are made of, and therefore, what we metabolize from food. It is our digestive system and functions. Earth is also where we "compost" and predigest some of our waste in our lymphatic system.

Earth is manifested here and now, and its energy is preponderant during the harvest season and during the time of transition between seasons.

The Earth Principle

Earth is. It is that place of stillness between Yin and Yang, the center of the cosmic wheel of eternal motion. Earth is here and now, the present moment, neither in the past nor in the future, but here and now in the eternity of the present. Earth, like heaven, is an absolute. In the I'Ching, it is represented by Absolute Yin in the Earth trigram (see Figure 7). Earth is then understood as the ultimate Yin power of existence that binds the universe together. It is the power that holds and harmonizes everything together from the molecular level to the realm of stars, planets, and galaxies. This is the power of gravity that no one and nothing can escape, the same power that gives us the feeling of falling, yet of being supported at the same time. Without it, we would all float off the planet and be lost in space without any support or connection.

When our Earth Chi is harmonious and healthy, we feel supported by existence, and generally feel confident, at ease, and comfortable with life. Solidly anchored in pragmatic reality, we are practical and find it easy to be present, free, receptive, and accepting.

When our Earth Chi is out of balance, we feel ungrounded, uprooted, never satisfied, always in doubt, and do not even trust ourselves. Because of this, it is easy for us to feel abandoned, out of place, awkward, self-conscious, and ill at ease.

Earth gives birth to Metal, controls Water, and is under the dominion of Wood.

In Earth, we find our common sense.

Mental aspects: practical, clever, spontaneous, conciliatory, sympathetic, able to see the whole picture.

Positive emotional qualities and feelings: fair, spontaneous, genuine, harmonious, elegant, practical, centered, rooted, stable, consistent, regular, balanced, vigorous, sympathetic, solid, satisfied, on time, in tune, synchronized, sociable, hospitable, nurturing, supportive, conciliatory, comfortable.

Negative emotional qualities and feelings: prejudiced, biased, cheating, lethargic, artificial, unfair, awkward, imbalanced, inconsistent, shaky, envious, disproportionate, unsynchronized, unfriendly, inhospitable, anxious, worried, blaming, judgmental, dissatisfied.

Earth symptoms: hypoglycemia, diabetes, inability to be on time (too early or too late), irregularity of meals in particular, overweight or underweight, water retention or over-dryness.

Power animal: Old Chinese Taoist tradition gives the Earth power to the pheasant, a beautiful and tasty fowl that prefers the comfort of earth rather than the vastness of the sky. So Earth manifests in such birds as the chicken, quail, and turkey. In other traditions, we find the cow, buffalo, pig, bear, and elephant, all very earthy animals.

Arts: pottery, weaving, all artisan crafts in general (knitting, shoemaking, furniture building, clothing—though not for fashion, which would be Metal), engineering and architecture, gardening and landscaping, cooking and all culinary arts, and everything connected with domesticity.

Occupations: engineering, architecture, crafts, farming, the food and hospitality industry.

Language: movement.

~~~~~~

Harmonizing Our Inner Earth Meditation

For this meditation, it is of the utmost importance that you feel comfortable. Do whatever it takes to sit in a comfortable location and position; disconnect your phone, and take your time.

- Sit comfortably and center your mind and your breath inside your abdomen behind your navel. Feel free to move and change your sitting position to feel more comfortable at any time during the meditation.

- Feel the support of the earth beneath you. Let the weight of your body sink as you inhale and push your weight comfortably down into the earth as you exhale. Feel the pushing back of that support from the earth and take in that feeling of unconditional support deep within you.

- Between your eyes, picture a big smile and a bright golden light—very bright, very golden, like the sun shining on a field of California poppies.

- Let the smile and the golden light become very bright and vivid between your eyes. Then bring them inside your mouth and let your entire mouth relax and smile. Feel like you just put something very good, very satisfying, in your mouth, and take the time to feel it expanding there.

- Next, swallow that good feeling of satisfaction and let it slowly spread through your entire digestive tract, from your mouth, throat, esophagus, stomach, intestines, all the way to your rectum. Let it harmonize all the digestive functions in your pancreas and liver.

- From your digestive system, feel that golden light and big smile spreading and nourishing all your muscles in your body. Feel all your muscles relaxing, smiling, gently stretching and turning bright golden, like getting a nice tan. Feel a sense of ease and satisfaction spreading to all your muscles and visualize that sense also spreading to your lymphatic system, flushing it with a sense of vigor.

- Feel all the attributes of Earth and feed your system with them: solidity, consistency, balance, harmony, nurturing, satisfaction, validation, support, comfort.

- In front of you, you are going to summon your ideal place on earth. The place where you feel in harmony, where you can be yourself completely, unconditionally accepted, validated, supported, nurtured, where you feel beautiful and at peace. It can be a place from the past or future, it could be a place where you have been or a completely imaginary place. Let it become very detailed and vivid right in front of you.

- Draw that idealized Earth energy to you. Absorb its power through your muscles, through your stomach, and taste it in your mouth. Feel your entire self there and how it feels inside your body. Let a sense of satisfaction and solidity permeate your whole being.

- Now you feel that sense of ease, solidity, unconditional support, and satisfaction with the bright golden light and the big smile through your whole being. Take the time to enjoy it, take the time to get used to it as something not only normal but indispensable.

· Keep the memory of this meditation deep within you.

Being in Touch with Breath and the Elemental Force of Metal

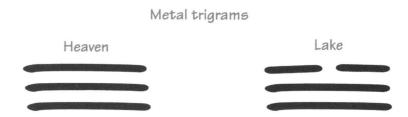

Metal trigrams

Heaven   Lake

Figure 8.
Heaven and Lake
trigrams

Deep in earth resides Metal, the most intriguing of the elements. In contrast to Wood, Metal is the cooling phase between Fire and Water, from the fruiting phase to maturation and a fall to the ground to liberate the seed. In contrast further to Wood, Metal is the nonrational, emotional phase that leads us in dreamtime and fantasy.

The Metal Principle

Metal represents the entire cooling-down phase from extreme Yang to extreme Yin, from Fire to Water. It is everything that condenses, concentrates, retracts, precipitates, conserves, shrinks, and freezes. It is the symbol of refinement and presentation (cosmetics, grooming, manicuring, wrapping), perfecting and finishing (polishing, shining), cutting (knife, sword, scissors), selecting, separating the good from the bad, reflection (mirror), and sensitivity (fur and skin). It is also the phase of decay from fruit (Earth) to the freeing of the seed (Water).

Metal is the surface tension between the elements such as water and air at the surface of the lake, and manifests inside our bodies through our system of skin and fasciae—the connective tissue that separates and wraps all the different organs, muscles, and muscle fibers down to the cellular level. It is an unbroken connection that runs uninterrupted from the depth of our bones to the surface of our skin. Our meridian system flows through this system, carrying our vital Chi to every cell, every tissue, and every organ. It is said that if we emptied our bodies of all tissues and kept only our system of fasciae, our mothers would still recognize us. Our system of fasciae holds our shape and form with all the information and energy dictated by our morphogenic field.[9]

According to Traditional Chinese Medicine, Metal power resides in the Lungs (Yin Metal organ) and is directed by the Large Intestine, the organ of elimination (Yang Metal organ). Metal thus affects our ability to breathe and to eliminate. It is our ability to differentiate what we need from what we don't. It enables us to breathe in essential elements such as oxygen and beneficial particles of flower essences and other fragrances, and breathe out nonessentials from the air such as carbon dioxide, toxic fumes, and whatever constitutes our body's exhaust. It is the power of elimination that uses our lungs to breathe out everything we don't need, and our large intestine to expel the by-products of our digestion.

Metal is the western direction (sunset) and the fall season.

Metal is the force of refinement given by heaven.

Like earth, heaven is an absolute: Absolute Yang. It is nonlocal and nontemporal—the absolute source of energy and information from which the Yang power arises. In this universe of Tai-Chi, heaven hides within Metal, inside the mirror of the Lake trigram (see Figure 8).

More so than the other elemental forces of nature, *Metal is the symbol of alchemy, ingenuity, and refinement.* Metal is not naturally found in nature ready to use. Metal first needs to be extracted, refined, forged, molded, shaped, and then sharpened and polished in order to be used to its fullest potential.

Metal is the power of the blade that can cut right through things cleanly. It is very sharp, very polished, very shiny, and very smooth. Metal is also the power of the mirror that reflects perfectly. The sword and the knife are not only weapons: throughout history, knives and swords have been worn more as decoration and signs of social status and male pride rather than as actual weapons. The majority of cultures worldwide often use a sword or a knife in rituals to manifest the integrity of the spirit and clarity of the soul. Myths abound with magic swords and mirrors, the sword's Yin counterpart. Metal is the power of elegance, grooming, and cosmetics, the power of appearance, of looks and presentation. It is a very Yin power, so it might not seem that important to the pragmatic Yang person, but it is certainly essential in all aspects of life at a very deep level for everyone.

Alchemy is popularly believed to be the practice of transforming base metal into gold. Just a few hundred years ago, a mere speck in the history of humanity, blacksmiths the world over were the wise men, the erudites, and the scientists of their times. Often, they were also priests or shamans, the messengers between heaven and earth, presiding over ceremonies and rituals. They spent their lives trying to find new ways to forge and perfect new alloys for greater sharpness and better luster. They did this not just by thinking, but also by pounding the metal and enduring the heat of their crucible and forge.

Taken as a metaphor for self-cultivation, however, internal alchemy refers to the process of transmuting and refining our body's energy. What is the energetic difference between base metal and gold? Base metal conducts energy with great difficulty; most of the energy is lost as heat. That's how an electric heater works: electricity is run through a piece of metal that cannot efficiently carry the amount of electricity sent through it, so it heats up. However, if it overheats, it burns out. To carry a large amount of electrical power, we need a better conductor. Copper does a good job of conducting a large amount of electricity compared to lesser metals, but gold is the best conductor. Even though gold is heavy, it takes only a minute amount of gold to carry a large amount of electricity, which is why it is commonly used in spacecraft. Applied to the human body, the alchemical practices of Chi-Kung and meditation allow us to cultivate and refine our bodies in order to be able to carry a greater and better grade of Chi—literally, changing our base metal into gold means being able to carry a higher grade of energy and information without burnout. The work of internal alchemy is aimed at refining our base existence into a better, more humane condition.

Metal is a powerful force in our life.

Metal carries the power of smoothness, sharpness, and trends; it is the "cool" power. It is the power for certain needs that cannot be explained: the power of order, esthetics, and cleanliness, beyond practicality—the power that makes us crazy over a stain on a shirt or a scratch on a brand new car. Even though the car runs fine, the scratch is always in our mind. There is nothing wrong with the car; it is just that it is scratched. People will understand if we decide to trade in our new car for one with no scratch. Such is the power of Metal.

In the I'Ching, Metal is represented by Lake, the mirror of the quiet lake that perfectly reflects the surrounding landscape. It is also the unpredictable and bottomless stormy lake, the power of the unconscious.

First and foremost, *Metal is our breath,* the ability to "cut" through air and separate oxygen from everything else. Breath is the bridge that connects and differentiates all levels of awareness: physical, mental, emotional, and spiritual. Breath is largely autonomic, nonconscious. Fortunately, we don't need to remember to breathe all the time, as this is automatically taken care of by part of us that has been very well trained over thousands of years of evolution. Feelings are proportional to our ability to breathe. The reason you and I don't breathe the same way is because we don't feel the same way. To be able to spontaneously breathe fully means that we are emotionally in touch with ourselves. It also means that if we don't breathe fully, we have no way of knowing whether or not we are in touch. We won't even know whether we are breathing fully until someone points it out to us. As far as we are concerned, we are "just fine" or we even "feel great." However, we are actually not feeling a thing! Not being able to feel is the origin of depression, which is not being able to feel the joys of life. Depression is the constant message we send ourselves: "If I can't enjoy life, I don't deserve to live!"

In our breath, we find the well-trained guardian that we mentioned in Chapter 1. The guardian, our denial system, won't prevent us from knowing about things that would be too painful to be aware of, but it protects the innocent and weak child within us from the horrors of traumatic events and emotional distress. The guardian also lets us know when we are old enough, wise enough, and possess a better support system and the emotional maturity necessary to deal with such trauma and stress. "Messages" from our guardian commonly take the form of repeated messages from our bodies such as chronic symptoms or frequent "accidents."

Within our breath, we hold the lock and the key to our healing process.

With Metal, we "get in touch," and we make contact not only with ourselves, but also with others. Breath is very important in communication. Sometimes we don't get along with certain people we meet for the first time just because our breath is "out of sync" with the other's. All the greeting rituals around the world have something in common: They force us to stop and synchronize our breath. Greetings are very important because they harmonize our energies even when we don't have anything to say to each other. Communication then happens at a much deeper and primal level, especially when we don't speak the same language.

Metal is also our ability to "be in touch," to communicate and feel. It is the power of sensitivity that controls the domain of emotions, our ability to know them, to feel them, and to differentiate them from thoughts and fantasies. It is the power of honesty, uprightness, and pride. The support of the entire five-element cycle is necessary for us to have full power in Metal. It takes all of the will of Water, the ingenuity of Wood, the spirit of Fire, and the unconditional support of Earth to have the power of honesty in Metal. Honesty takes strength and wisdom, and that's why it is difficult to find.

Metal is also very "touchy," very capricious. This nonrationality of Metal is very hard to take for the rationally oriented Wood personality. I have friends very different than I am with different ideas, different lifestyles, and different political views, but when we get together we have a great time even if we make fun of each other's differences! Other people I know have the same views I do. We have much in common; we care for the same things and are involved in very similar activities. Somehow, though, it doesn't really "click" between us, and sometimes we can barely stand each other. This is the mystery of relationship. It is irrational; it can't even be discussed. It's just the way we feel! The I'Ching describes this in the universal laws of attraction, repulsion, and indifference. It says specifically that there is no such thing as being liked by everyone. There will always be someone to hate us no matter what, as there will always be someone to love us no matter what, and some people will be completely indifferent. These indifferent people won't even notice us because, for them, we won't even exist! For no other reason than just because! That's the way things are—the way the world is.

When Metal Chi is abundant, we get in touch very easily with ourselves and with others. We have a very precise sense of how other people feel, and how we feel. Being true to our feelings, we have the courage to own them. This is the power of honesty.

When our Metal Chi becomes deficient, we lose touch. We lose our ability to know our feelings and are unable to care about the feelings of others. Not being able to feel, then, leads us into a state of depression sometimes so deep that we are not even aware of being unhappy. We just don't feel!

Metal feeds Water, cuts Wood, and is under the control of Fire.

In Metal, we find our soul.

Mental aspects: refinement, sensitivity to emotions.

Positive emotional qualities and feelings: sensitive, honest, courageous, cool, firm, proud, uplifted, resonant, pure, pardoning, forgiving, cultivated, refined, faithful, loyal.

Negative emotional qualities and feelings: reactive, hypocritical, cowardly, hesitant, treacherous, deceitful, sad, depressed, tedious, confused, unreliable, irresponsible, petty, jealous, resentful.

Metal symptoms: skin problems (rashes), elimination problems, breathing problems, very white complexion.

Power animal: The white tiger is also represented by all felines in general, and is very powerful, unpredictable, playful, dangerous, sensual, sensitive, capricious, nonrational, cool, smooth, and beautiful.

Arts: music, the art of summoning feelings from pure abstraction, the power of sophistication from simple, practical lines (Japanese Zen style) to gaudy, rococo, and naïve childlike style.

Occupations: All activities related to the shape and form of things (fashion, design, cosmetics), activities connected with attractiveness such as publicity and advertisement, perfumes, auto design, interior decorating, furniture, antiques, landscaping.

Language: feelings.

Inner Metal Meditation: Lung Healing Chi-Kung

- Sit comfortably with your back erect but not stiff.

- Center your breath behind your navel. Visualize and feel an empty sphere behind your navel. Feel that sphere expanding as you inhale and shrinking back as you exhale.

- Guide each in-breath toward your pelvic floor and sacrum and up to your shoulder blades simultaneously.

- Feel the support of the earth beneath you through the chair or whatever you are sitting on. Let the weight of your body sink as you inhale, and push your weight comfortably down as you exhale. Feel the support from the earth and take in that feeling of unconditional support deep within you. Use that feeling to make yourself feel more comfortable, better supported, and more solid.

- Keep breathing toward your pelvic floor and sacrum and up to your shoulder blades, and between your eyes picture a big smile and a bright white light—very bright, very white, like the sun shining on a blanket of newly fallen snow.

- Take the time to observe that bright white light with the big smile on it. Make it very real, very clear, and very distinct right between your eyes.

- Bring that bright white light and the smile to your nose and breathe them inside your lungs.

- Let the bright white light and the smile expand to the whole volume of your lungs, to your windpipe, all the bronchiae and alveolae of your lungs, and through the whole surface of your diaphragm. Smile in them.

- If you have any dark spots in your lungs, or any place in your lungs where you have a hard time feeling or visualizing, flash the bright white light there.

- Smile in your lungs. Smile in your diaphragm. Smile everywhere your breath takes you.

- In front of you, visualize a perfect representation of Metal's alchemical force: a beautiful mountain lake at the foot of a high crest at a high altitude—a very distant and inaccessible lake, under a deep blue sky.

- Look at the lake. It is deep, formed from pure and cold glacial mountain water such as you can only find at high altitudes in remote places.

- It is a very quiet, very calm lake, with a smooth surface reflecting the surrounding landscape perfectly like a clean mirror. Look inside the depth of it. You can see very deep and far through the crystalline water. It is deep and clear; it seems bottomless.

· Keep that beautiful archetypal representation of the lake right in front of you. Breathe in deeply and be aware of your own inner Metal—your lungs, your diaphragm, and the whole surface of your skin. Be aware of how they feel—the breath in your lungs, the expansion of your diaphragm, the feeling of your skin.

· Then, be aware of your own private inner mountain lake. Feel the energy from your lungs, and picture it as a lake inside your chest.

· Take the time to really feel your inner lake clearly and accurately rather than imagining an ideal lake. The lake you have inside is very real and very meaningful. How does your lake feel? Is it a quiet lake, or is it a stormy lake? Is the sun shining, or is it foggy and hard to see?

· Think of how you would describe your inner lake. How big is it? How deep is the bottom? What is the bottom made of? Clean rock, or mud? How clear is the water?

· What else is in the lake? Is there any life? Algae, plants, fish, creatures hiding at the bottom?

· Is there anything you don't like in your lake? Is there anything that would prevent you from diving in and swimming in your lake? Is it too deep, or not deep enough? Too muddy? Or are you just afraid?

· Stay with that feeling for a while and breathe through it. Breathe deeply but gently.

· It is okay to look at the depth of the lake. Take a nice long look inside your lake until the mud settles at the bottom and the water gets progressively clearer.

· Slowly you are able to see more deeply into the water. It is okay, there is fresh water running from deep wells at the bottom of the lake.

· Yes, there are shapes; yes, there are things you don't like to look at there, but it is okay. They are there anyway; you might as well look at them.

- No need to understand, no need to justify, no need for explanation, or looking for alternatives or solutions. Just get in touch with the feelings associated with these visions and the familiarity of these feelings.

- Keep breathing deeply and give yourself permission to be as abstract and non-rational as possible. Without labeling them, be aware of any familiarity you have with these feelings. Stay with the way they feel rather than trying to understand or interpret them.

- Be aware of the lake being in your chest, being in your lungs. Be aware of the smoke in your lungs, the cough, the asthma being the mud, the turbidity.

- Breathe slowly and deeply, expanding your breath to your pelvic floor, to your tailbone, and all the way up your back to your shoulder blades.

- Breathe deeply in your abdomen until you start feeling coolness, perhaps even cold, coming from your body.

- Feel different waves of cold moving out of your body and let your body react and move on its own. You might feel your jaws shaking, your feet and your legs wanting to move and stretch. Follow the movement of your pelvis and your spine without trying to understand the significance of anything. Let the energy flow through you.

- Push your feet into the ground to get good support from the earth's energy and a good grounding connection. (If you are lying down, raise your knees with your feet flat on the ground.)

- If the cold and body movements are bearable, continue and let the cold waves clear up as you visualize your inner lake in your lungs becoming clearer and cleaner.

- If the cold and body spasms are too intense and unpleasant, give yourself permission to bear them for a while, and liberate the cold from the depth of your lower abdomen in successive waves while breathing more deeply. Then slow down, but don't stop. You are almost there!

- Next, be aware of your inner lake in your chest and summon again that beautiful archetypal lake in front of you, the most beautiful lake on earth.

- Draw in the energy from the outside lake to your inner lake and feel your inner lake growing deeper, clearer, and fresher.

- Feel the muddiness disappearing. Feel the oppressive feelings lifting off of your chest and dissipating from your body.

- Feel the power of the archetypal lake within you: the beauty, the clarity, the cleanliness, the reflection of the landscape on the mirror of the lake inside your chest.

- Smell the mountain air, very pure, very crisp. Feel the coolness in your chest from a solid and clear pair of lungs.

- Keep the memory of this practice deep within you.

Stay connected with any emotional insights that might come up during this practice, and others. The safety valves are open, and there is no regression possible. Your body will continue to release, especially at night during sleep and dreamtime. Make sure you provide the space and time for it. Go to bed early and sleep by yourself until you feel fine. As with any *Healing from Within* practice, it is better to practice less intensely, but more often until the discomfort disappears.

Be careful about driving. After your practice, take a short, leisurely walk, finishing with a bit of brisk walking. Then you'll be ready for driving.

The Ba-Gua of Later Heaven
representing life and the three dimensional manifestations of the universe (Tai-Chi)

Color code: Fire Water Wood Metal Earth

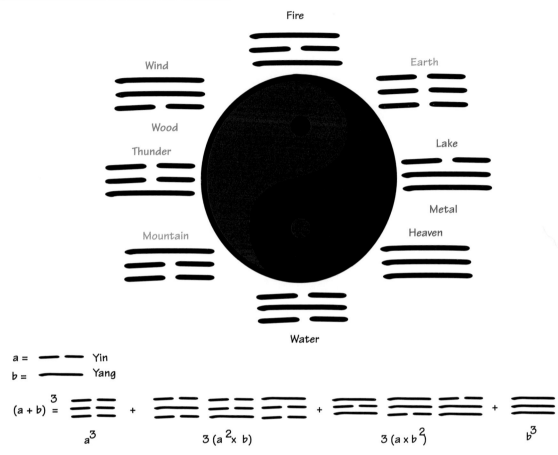

$a =$ — — Yin

$b =$ ——— Yang

$(a + b)^3 =$ [hexagram symbols] $+$ [hexagram symbols] $+$ [hexagram symbols] $+$ [hexagram symbols]

a^3 $3(a^2 \times b)$ $3(a \times b^2)$ b^3

(From "The Great Tao", Dc. Stephen T. Chang, San Francisco, Tao publishing, 1985)

Water: extreme Yin for attention, alertness and being essential

Fire: extreme Yang for clarity and being consistent

Earth: absolute Yin for great flexibility and following

Mountain: Earth attributes of solidity and stability

Thunder: Wood attributes for creative energy and inner silence

Wind: Wood attributes for penetrating power and going deep

Lake: Metal attributes of playfulness and lightness of being

Heaven: Metal attributes for absolute Yang, constant improvement and evolution

The 10,000 Things are the infinite possibilities of all the manifestations of life put in the perspective of the 8 tendencies formed by the 5 Elements of life. When multiplied by itself, reminiscent of the double helix of the DNA, the 8 tendencies rise to the 64 hexagrams of the I'ching. Notice the motion of Tai-Chi given by the opposite forces of Yin and Yang, Water and Fire, Wood and Metal along the Earth axis of Earth-Mountain. Notice also that the orientation of the elements corresponds to the location of the vital organs in the body: Fire/heart on top, Water/genitals at the bottom, Wood/liver on the right (rational side), Metal/lungs on the left (sentimental side), Earth/pancreas on the upper left.

**Plate 1: The Ba-Gua of Later Heaven, representing life
and the three-dimensional manifestations of the universe (Tai-Chi)**

Taoist Cosmology

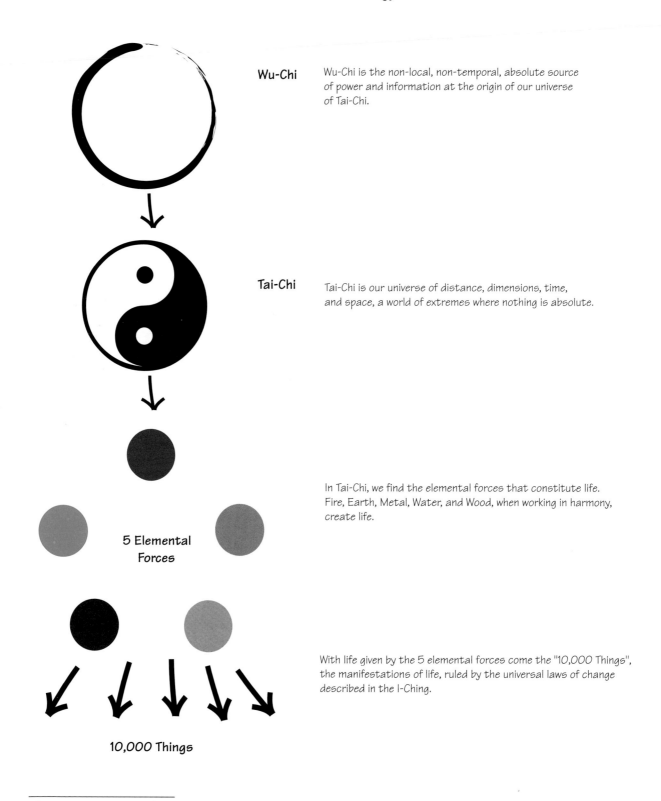

Wu-Chi

Wu-Chi is the non-local, non-temporal, absolute source of power and information at the origin of our universe of Tai-Chi.

Tai-Chi

Tai-Chi is our universe of distance, dimensions, time, and space, a world of extremes where nothing is absolute.

In Tai-Chi, we find the elemental forces that constitute life. Fire, Earth, Metal, Water, and Wood, when working in harmony, create life.

5 Elemental Forces

With life given by the 5 elemental forces come the "10,000 Things", the manifestations of life, ruled by the universal laws of change described in the I-Ching.

10,000 Things

Plate 2: Taoist Cosmology

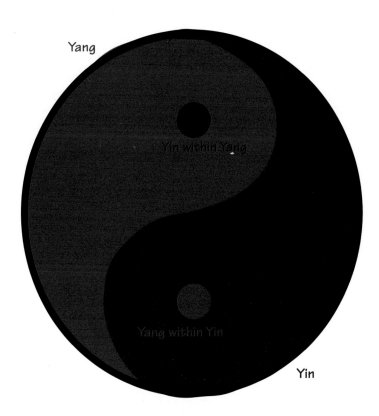

Tai-Chi

Yang

Yin within Yang

Yang within Yin

Yin

This symbol is the representation of our universe, the universe of space and time, dualities and opposites. It consists of three dimensions represented by the opposites Yin and Yang and the force that holds them together (the black circle around Yin and Yang). In Tai-Chi, we find extremes but no absolute: at the extreme Yang, we find Yin within Yang, and at the extreme Yin, we find Yang within Yin.

Tai-Chi comes out of Wu-Chi, which means no Chi, no life, nothingness. But in that nothingness reside all the information and energy for the creation of our universe. So we say that Wu-Chi is the force of creation, the Creator, or God. In this universe of Tai-Chi, Chi is the energy and the information that give life. Chi is the breath of God.

Plate 3: Tai-Chi

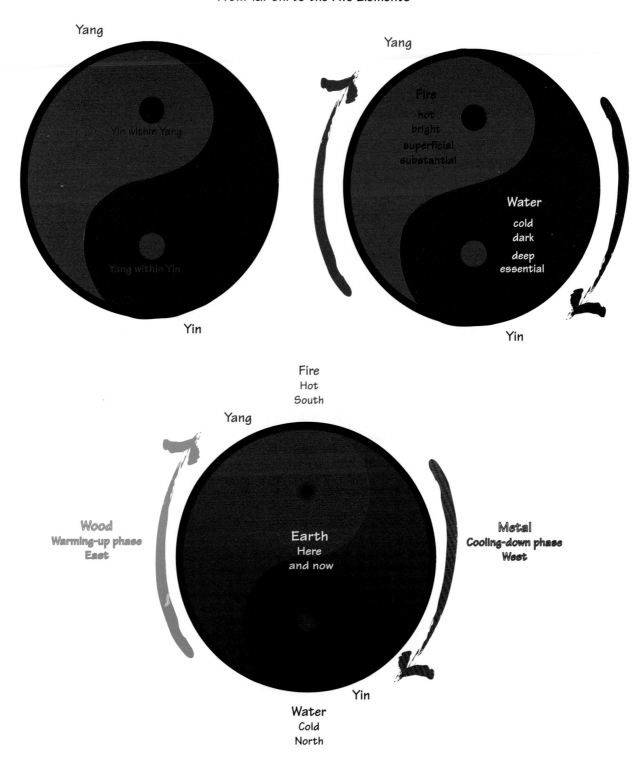

Plate 4: From Tai-Chi to the Five Elements

**Location of the Earth
Elemental Force**

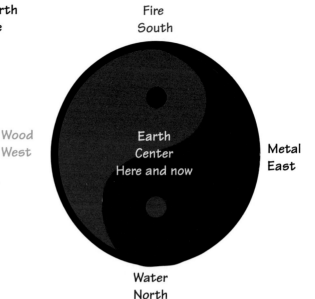

Earth is at the center of the universe. It is gravity, the power of here and now that binds everything together from celestial bodies down to the atoms and their electrons. In the cycle of a year, the time the earth takes to circle the sun, the moon circles the earth 13 times - 13 moons or 13 months. There are 4 seasons of 3 months of 28 days forming the 12 months of the 4 seasons. Plus one additional month made of the week of transition (Earth) in between each season.

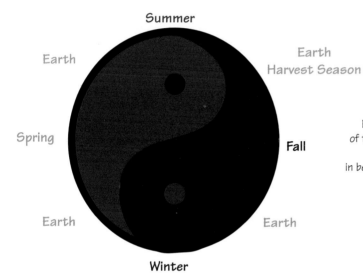

Earth is the 13th month of the lunar year comprised of the week of transition in between the 4 usual seasons.

However, the Earth Force principles of nurturing, comfort and harmony are preponderant during the Harvest Season, or Indian Summer, a fifth season in between Summer and Fall; thus, the Earth location came to be in between Fire and Metal. However, it is often useful to remember that Earth is the time of transition in between any phases and all seasons.

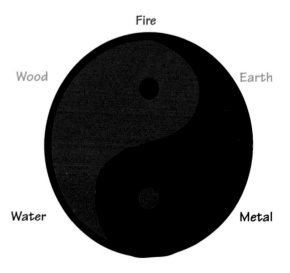

Plate 5: Location of the Earth elemental force

Law of Creation

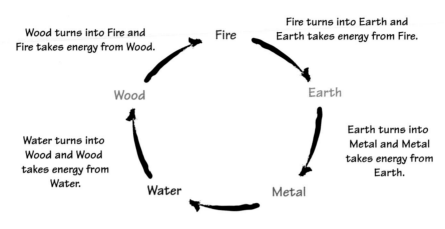

Wood turns into Fire and Fire takes energy from Wood.

Fire turns into Earth and Earth takes energy from Fire.

Water turns into Wood and Wood takes energy from Water.

Earth turns into Metal and Metal takes energy from Earth.

Metal turns into Water and Water takes energy from Metal.

Plate 6: The law of creation

Law of Control
or Preservation of the Elemental Forces

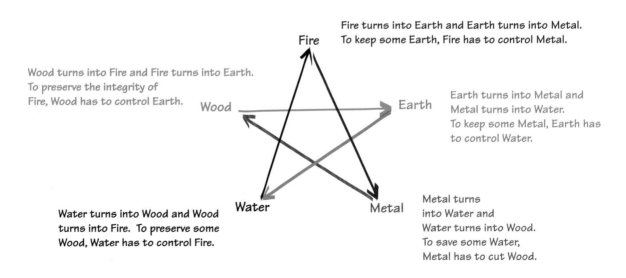

Fire turns into Earth and Earth turns into Metal. To keep some Earth, Fire has to control Metal.

Wood turns into Fire and Fire turns into Earth. To preserve the integrity of Fire, Wood has to control Earth.

Earth turns into Metal and Metal turns into Water. To keep some Metal, Earth has to control Water.

Water turns into Wood and Wood turns into Fire. To preserve some Wood, Water has to control Fire.

Metal turns into Water and Water turns into Wood. To save some Water, Metal has to cut Wood.

Plate 7: The law of control, or preservation of the elemental forces

Law of Overpowering and Surrendering

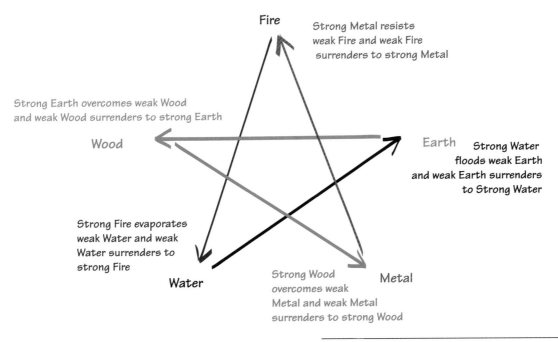

Fire

Strong Metal resists weak Fire and weak Fire surrenders to strong Metal

Strong Earth overcomes weak Wood and weak Wood surrenders to strong Earth

Wood

Earth

Strong Water floods weak Earth and weak Earth surrenders to Strong Water

Strong Fire evaporates weak Water and weak Water surrenders to strong Fire

Water

Strong Wood overcomes weak Metal and weak Metal surrenders to strong Wood

Metal

Plate 8: Law of overpowering and surrendering

The Five Elemental colors and tastes within Tai-Chi

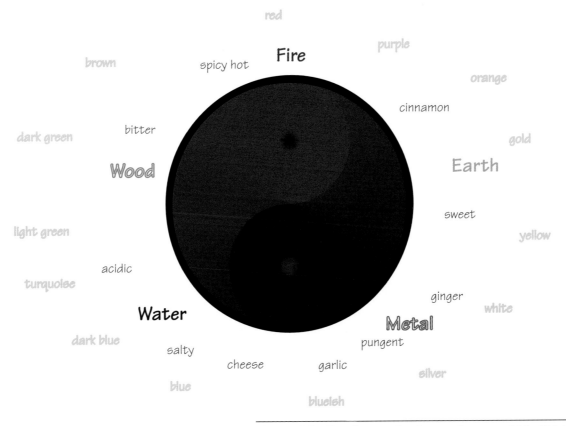

red

brown

spicy hot

Fire

purple

orange

cinnamon

dark green

bitter

Wood

gold

Earth

sweet

light green

yellow

turquoise

acidic

dark blue

Water

ginger

white

Metal

blue

salty

pungent

cheese

garlic

silver

blueish

Plate 9: The five elemental colors and tastes within Tai-Chi

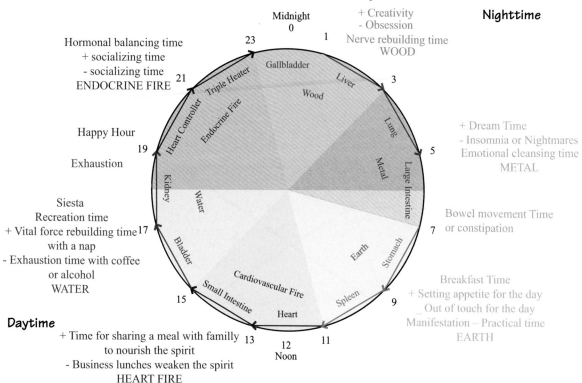

Behavior and the time of day

- The Chi inside the meridian system ebbs and flows like a tide following the progression of the sun. Thus, the meridian system follows the order of basic daily needs and habits.
- **If you stand with your arms stretched over your head:**
Yang meridians: go down from hands to head and from head to feet
Yin meridians: go up from feet to chest and from chest to hands
- The 12 meridians, in a 24-hour period, form 3 loops of 2 pairs of meridians (Yin & Yang), each loop covering an 8-hour period.

The daytime loop
Earth meridians:
7:00 a.m. to 9:00 a.m.: Yang Earth, Stomach meridians, from face to second toes.
9:00 a.m. to 11:00 a.m.: Yin Earth, Spleen-Pancreas meridians, from the big toes to the sides of the chest.
Cardio-Vascular Fire meridians
11:00 a.m. to 1:00 p.m.: Yin Cardio-Vascular Fire, Heart meridians, from the chest to the little fingers.
1:00 p.m. to 3:00 p.m.: Yang Cardio-Vascular Fire, Small Intestine meridians, from the little fingers to both sides of the face.

The evening loop
Water meridians
3:00 p.m. to 5:00 p.m.: Yang Water, Bladder meridians from the corners of the eyes, up the forehead and down the back to the little toes.
5:00 p.m. to 7:00 p.m.: Yin Water, Kidney meridians, from the bottom of the feet, up the inside of the legs, up to the collarbone.
Endocrine Fire meridians
7:00 p.m. to 9:00 p.m.: Yin Endocrine Fire, Heart Controller meridians, from both armpits to the middle fingers.
9:00 p.m. to 11:00 p.m.: Yang Endocrine Fire, Triple Heater meridians, from the ring fingers to the sides of the head by the ears.

The nighttime loop
Wood meridians
11:00 p.m. to 1:00 a.m.: Yang Wood, Gallbladder meridians, from both sides of the cranium down the sides of the body to the fourth toes.
1:00 a.m. to 3:00 a.m.: Yin Wood, Liver meridians, from the big toes to the chest.
Metal meridians
3:00 a.m. to 5:00 a.m.: Yin Metal, Lung meridians, from the chest to the thumbs.
5:00 a.m. to 7:00 a.m.: Yang Metal, Large Intestine meridians, from the index fingers to the opposite sides of the nose.

Plate 10: Behavior and the time of day

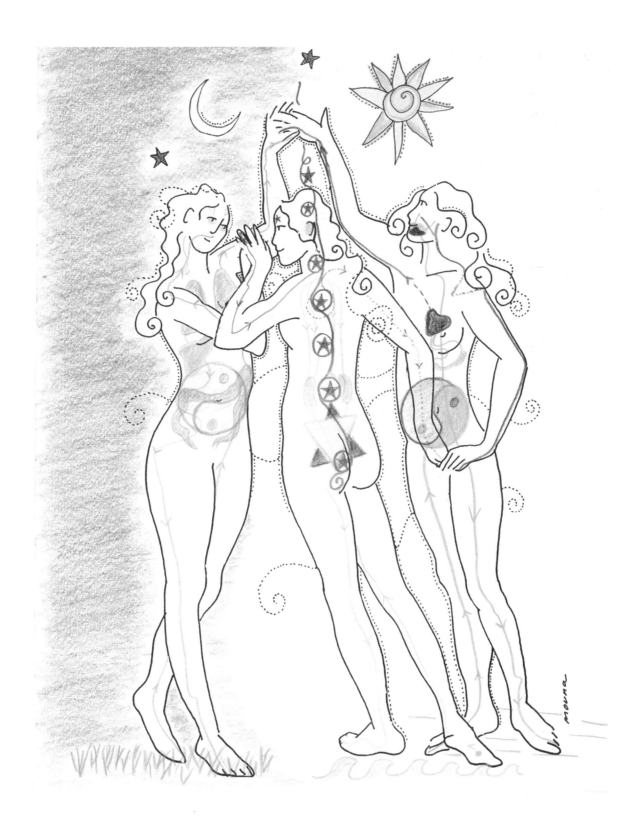

Plate 11: The three meridian loops and time of day

The daytime loop

Within the daytime loop of the meridian system is the Earth meridian system. Stomach, from 7:00 a.m. to 9:00 a.m., runs from both sides of the face to the second toes, and Spleen-Pancreas, from 9:00 a.m. to 11:00 a.m., goes up the body from the big toes to the spleen and pancreas at the sides of the chest. The Cardio-Vascular Fire meridian system includes Heart, from 11:00 a.m. to 1:00 p.m., which stretches from the heart and the chest to the little fingers, and Small Intestine, from 1:00 p.m. to 3:00 p.m., which goes from the little fingers to both sides of the face. Here the Cardio-Vascular Fire meridian system connects with the evening loop and the Bladder meridian.

The Earth force has the capacity to bind and harmonize. In the morning and midday hours, our Earth allows the creative Fire in our Spirit to create. Fire can thus safely warm us and cook for us under the protection of the hearth or the stove in our home, Therefore, each day we have the ability to be practical and productive, and to fulfill our life purpose.

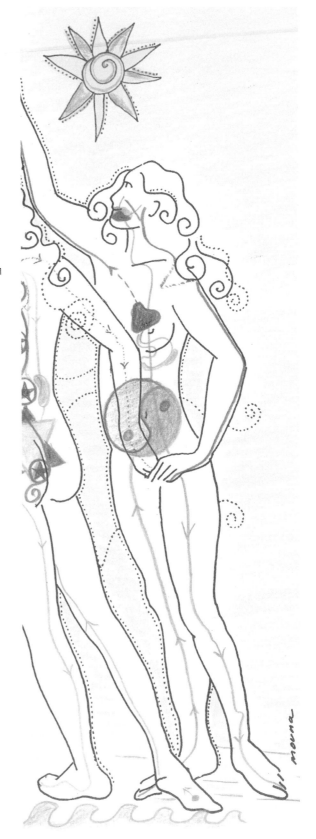

Plate 12: The daytime loop

The evening loop

The evening loop of the meridian system is composed of the Water meridian system. The Bladder meridian goes from 3:00 p.m. to 5:00 p.m. and stretches from the corners of the eyes, up the forehead and down the back to the little toes. The Kidney meridian goes from 5:00 p.m. to 7:00 p.m. reaching from the bottom of the feet, up the inside of the legs to the collar bones. The Endocrine Fire meridian system with the Heart Controller meridian goes from 7:00 p.m. to 9:00 p.m., stretching from both armpits to the middle fingers. The Triple Heater meridian is from 9:00 p.m. to 11:00 p.m. Reaching from the ring fingers to the sides of the head by the ears, it connects with the next loop and the Gallbladder meridian.

Water manifests in our genes, our culture, and our historical background. Endocrine Fire is our celestial fire, encompassing the evolution of human consciousness, which directs our spirit. The interaction of Water and Fire reproduces the marriage between Heaven and Earth, or more precisely, since planet Earth is already part of the heavens, between human consciousness and the world we have created. This is the best time for socializing, intimacy, and spirited conversations.

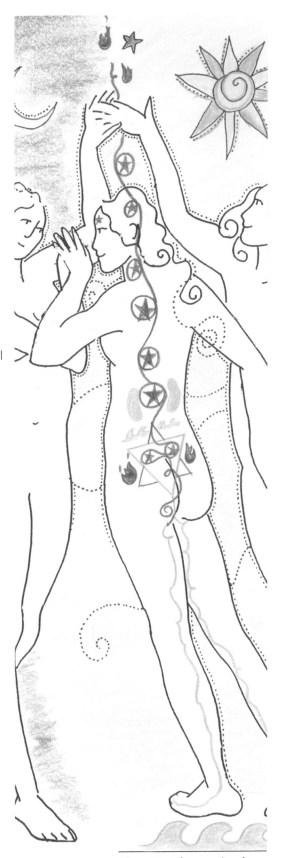

Plate 13: The evening loop

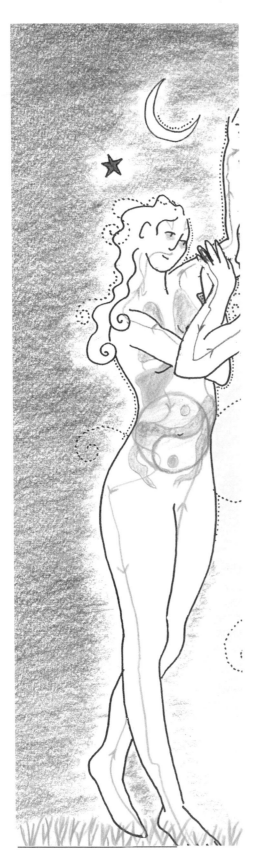

The nighttime loop

The nighttime loop includes the Wood meridian system. Gallbladder, lasting from 11:00 p.m. to 1:00 a.m., runs from both sides of the cranium down the sides of the body to the fourth toes. Liver, lasting from 1:00 a.m. to 3:00 p.m., runs from the big toes to the liver under the right ribcage and to both sides of the chest. Also part of the nighttime loop is the Metal meridian system. Lung, from 3:00 a.m. to 5:00 a.m., goes from the lungs to the thumbs, and Large Intestine, from 5:00 a.m. to 7:00 a.m., stretches from the index fingers to the opposite sides of the nose. This is where the nighttime loop connects with breathing and the lungs, as well as to the Stomach meridian and the daytime loop.

Wood and Metal are two complementary forces symbolized, respectively, by the Dragon and the White Tiger. They manifest as our rational thinking (Wood/Dragon) and our emotions (Metal/White Tiger). Mysterious forces rising from the darkness of night, they are ruled by the moon and stars, and interact in our dreams. The balance of Wood and Metal in our sleep determines our level of wakefulness, mental clarity, and emotional maturity. It also measures our mental health while we are awake.

Plate 14: The nighttime loop

The Seven Levels of Individuation

The seven levels of individuation correspond to the seven chakras of Ayurvedic tradition, the seven informational centers of the body influenced by our main endocrine glands.

The seventh level of individuation begins in the pineal gland and includes the whole endocrine system. It connects and aligns all the informational levels from the top of our head to the heavens above, down to our pelvic floor. The Earth, the underworld, and our ancestors move through these to give us guidance in life.

The sixth level of individuation is in our pituitary and pineal glands, mid-eyebrow and at the nape of our neck. They affect the brain and nervous system, determined introspection, and our capacity to connect, and to reconcile abstraction and rationality.

The fifth level of individuation, our thyroid, is in our throat and neck, where our capacity to express ourselves resides. This area also extends to our arms and hands, which allow us to reach out, to give, and to receive.

The fourth level of individuation is in our heart area, front and back, including our thymus gland. It relates to our spirit, what we hold within us that we need to manifest in our life.

The third level of individuation corresponding to our solar plexus, the 11th dorsal vertebra and diaphragm area, and to our pancreas. Our Earth center lets us know how we feel about ourselves and reflects our capacity to deal with periods of transition and change.

The second level of individuation corresponds to our adrenals: the kidneys, navel, and belt area. It corresponds to our genetic and cultural background and holds ancestral and atavistic influences.

The first level of individuation corresponds to our pelvic floor, sacrum, lower abdomen, and reproductive glands. The pelvic floor receives all the Earth attributes of unconditional support, nurturing, trust, and confidence in life. It is where we feel our sense of comfort or discomfort. The sacrum generates life momentum. The lower abdomen contains the sexual center from which the enjoyment of life is created.

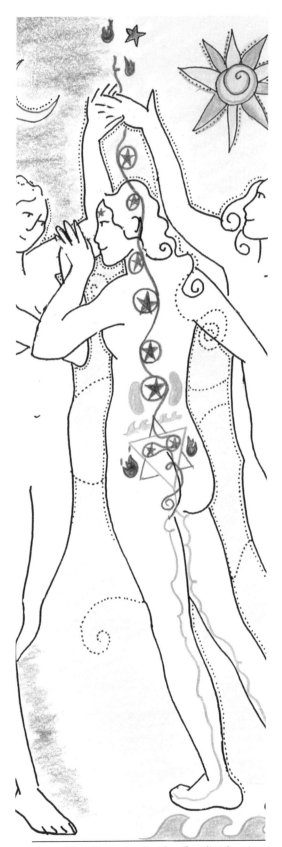

Plate 15: The seven levels of individuation

The Physical Aspects
of the Five-Element Organ System

The Five Elemental Forces manifest through the five metabolic functions that support life in the body. The Yin organs (capitalized) are in charge of the quality of Chi (Yin function). The Yang organs are in charge of the movement of Chi (Yang function). The main organs (not capitalized) gave their name to the Yin Function but have often other functions. The influenced tissues, the senses and the sense organs are the parts of the body affected by the quality of the Chi of each of the five metabolic functions.

The Fire element rules over two different systems: the cardio-vascular and the endocrine systems.

CARDIO-VASCULAR FIRE
Heart
Small intestine
heart and arteries
blood
tongue for good taste
(nourishes the spirit)

ENDOCRINE FIRE
Pericardium/Heart Controller
Triple Heater
endocrine glands
hormones
tongue for speech
(communication)

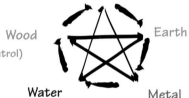

Liver
Gall-bladder
liver (blood filter
and storage, nerve control)
nerves
eyesight

Spleen - Pancreas
Stomach
pancreas - liver (digestion)
spleen (lymphatic - recycling waste)
muscles
mouth (for taste)

Kidney (DNA - genetic inheritance)
Bladder
kidneys (organs)
bone , marrow and teeth
hearing

Lung
Large Intestine
lungs (organs)
skin, epithelial tissue, fasciae
smell and touch

Every part of the human body is human, therefore, we cannot expect any part of us to react any differently than we would when put in the same situation. The mental, emotional, and physical processes are intimately interconnected and reflect on each other.

• **WATER:** When our Water system is overstressed we get fatigued and our kidneys can be affected as well as our ears, the health of our bones, gums and teeth. We then are easily afraid and lose creativity and drive. Conversely, long exposure to fear and fright can make us fatigued, weaken our kidneys, and negatively affect our bone density, our sense of hearing and the health of our teeth.

• **WOOD:** When our liver (Wood) is toxic we easily lose control of our nerves, we feel aggressive and angry and our vision acuity decreases. Being angry for a long period of time weakens our liver and can have the same effect as being intoxicated or poisoned; we lose our appetite and we can hardly digest our food and emotions.

• **FIRE:** Emotional stress affects our heart (Fire) and hormonal system (Endocrine Fire)increasing blood pressure, causing hormonal imbalance and headaches. A pressured heart makes us edgy and on the run, preventing us from being in touch with our spirit and emotions.

• **EARTH:** Our digestive system (Earth) can be affected by either a bad diet or a lack of comfort at home or at work. The worse we feel in our stomach, the more difficult it is to feel comfortable in life in general. We then lose our confidence, emotional balance and sense of trust.

• **METAL:** Weak lungs (Metal) bring a propensity for sorrow, nostalgia, and being taciturn. Extreme grief, especially when it is not validated, can cause great damage to our lungs, skin and colon, causing breathing problems, skin rashes and poor bowel movement.

Plate 16: The physical aspects of the five-element organ system

The Mental Aspects
of the Five-Element Organ System

When the Chi is abundant, harmonious, and flows healthily and unobstructed through our five internal organ systems, our five mental aspects unite to provide an enlightened perspective on life. When an organ system is impaired, it upsets the whole mental balance.

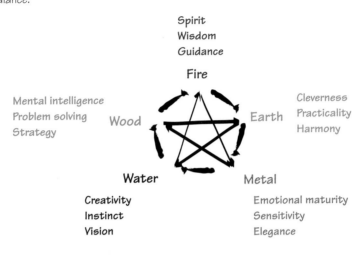

Plate 17: The mental aspects of the five-element organ system

The Emotional Aspects
of the Five-Element Organ System

Positive emotions: when Chi is healthy and abundant
Negative emotions: when Chi is restricted or corrupted

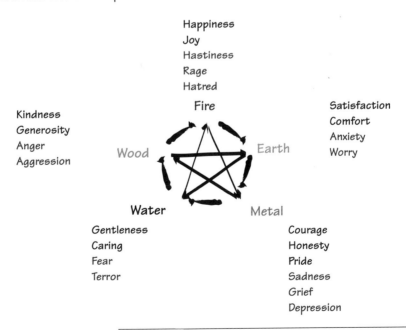

Plate 18: The emotional aspects of the five-element organ system

Positive and negative mental and emotional categories

From the Taoist perspective of the Five Elemental Forces, there are five categories of mental and emotional aspects corresponding to the quality of the Chi, the energy and information, associated with these mental and emotional aspects.

If the Chi is healthy and abundant the mental and emotional aspects tend toward the positive, and when the Chi is deficient or weak, these aspects tend toward the negative. From the Taoist perspective, and since we are talking about energy, there is no judgemental value to these words. The same way that there is nothing wrong with a negative pole of a battery and nothing particularly good about its positive pole , there is nothing wrong about negative emotions and nothing so good about positive emotions: when in danger, fear makes us run faster; when rich, we have to share so we won't rot with our excess wealth. Mental and emotional aspects are completely dependent on our physiological health. When our kidneys are weak, we are more fearful; when our digestive system is imbalanced, we feel more anxious; when our liver is toxic, we feel antagonistic; when pressure builds in our heart, we are insensitive and we become hasty; and when our lungs are hurt, we feel sad or melancholic.

Wood (positive)	Wood (negative)	Fire (positive)	Fire (negative)	Earth (positive)	Earth (negative)
Kind	Angry	High spirited	Hateful	Clever	Invasive
Generous	Vindictive	Wise	Superstitious	Practical	Abusive
Intelligent	Slanderer	Bright	Pretentious	Confident	Awkward
Humble	Traitor	Passionate	Dull	Reliable	Prejudiced
Tempered	Suspicious	Enthusiastic	Dispassionate	Reasonable	Unreliable
Pleasant	Stingy	Charismatic	No sense of humor	Fair	Biased
Cool-headed	Cunning	Spiritual	Mocking	Sensible	Fake
Discreet	Calculating	Joyful	Ridicule	Open-minded	Artificial
Relaxed	Loud	Happy	Dispirited	Authentic	Self-conscious
Soft	Conspicuous	Warm	Cold	Genuine	Ashamed
Clear-minded	Uptight	Virtuous	Ill-considered	Spontaneous	Guilty
Productive	Contolling	Respectful	Obsequious	Balanced	Imbalanced
Progressive	Hypervigilant	Grateful	Thoughtless	Centered	Not available
Cooperative	Obsessed	Loving	Vicious	Present	Flaky
Constructive	Compulsive	Patient	Cruel	Stable	Shaky
Conciliatory	Formalistic	Refined taste	Impatient	Dependable	Ill at ease
Team-spirited	Antagonistic		Tactless	Comfortable	Inconsiderate
	Aggressive			Nurturing	Greedy
	Argumentative			In-tune	glutton
	Competitive			On-time	Craving
				Synchronized	Possessive
				Harmonious	Envious
				Empathetic	Out of tune
				Adaptable	Desynchronized
				Convivial	Unfriendly
				Sociable	Inhospitable
				Hospitable	Selfish
					Intrusive

Water (positive)	Water (negative)	Metal (positive)	Metal (negative)
Calm	Agitated	Honest	Dishonest
Positive	Negative	Courageous	Deceitful
Strong-willed	Weak	Firm	Deceptive
Gentle	Rough	Frank	Hypocritical
Considerate	Inconsiderate	Hopeful	Tedious
Consistent	Rushed	Uplifted	Pedantic
Creative	Boring	Resonant	Formalistic
Innovative	Scattered	Mature	Irresponsible
Original	Liar	Forgiving	Unreliable
Traditional	Coward	Smooth	Rude
Protective	Destructive	Refined	Impolite
Conservative	Impulsive	Easy going	Hesitant
Encompassing	Fleeting	Affectionate	Prideless
Sensuous	Lewd	Polite	Affected
Sensual	Fearful	Proud	Low self-esteem
Clear	Scared	Elegant	Hopeless
Cool	Terrorized	In touch	Diconnected
	Paranoid	Sympathetic	Melancholic
			Sad

Plate 19: Positive and negative mental and emotional categories

Law of Creation

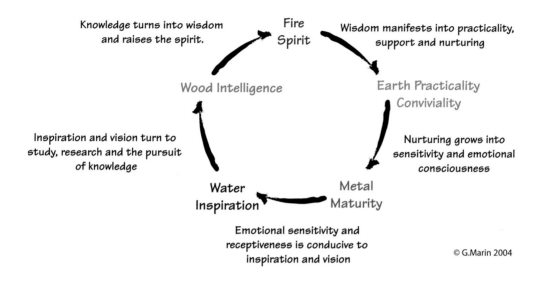

Knowledge turns into wisdom and raises the spirit.

Fire Spirit

Wisdom manifests into practicality, support and nurturing

Wood Intelligence

Earth Practicality Conviviality

Inspiration and vision turn to study, research and the pursuit of knowledge

Nurturing grows into sensitivity and emotional consciousness

Water Inspiration

Metal Maturity

Emotional sensitivity and receptiveness is conducive to inspiration and vision

© G.Marin 2004

Plate 20: Law of Creation

Law of Control

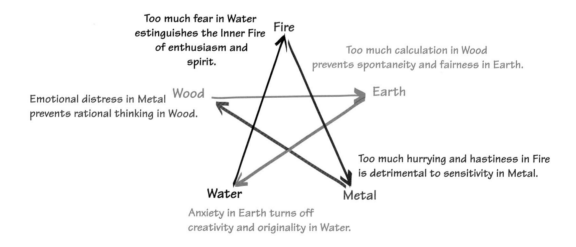

Too much fear in Water estinguishes the Inner Fire of enthusiasm and spirit.

Fire

Too much calculation in Wood prevents spontaneity and fairness in Earth.

Emotional distress in Metal prevents rational thinking in Wood.

Wood

Earth

Too much hurrying and hastiness in Fire is detrimental to sensitivity in Metal.

Water

Metal

Anxiety in Earth turns off creativity and originality in Water.

Plate 21: Law of Control

Taoist perspective on attitudes and reactions

The 5 element system allows for a wider perspective on human feelings and behavior. Each element represents tendencies. Furthermore, emotions are not as exclusive as thoughts: we all have, at any moment a whole spectrum of different emotions available while we can only think about one thing at a time. Thoughts require focus while emotions manifest in a wide range at any given moment. This explains the apparent contradictions between thinking, feeling, and behaving.

Practitioners of the healing arts have to learn these tendencies, be able to recognize them and be able to "juggle" with them to help their clients recognize their personal tendencies. Only then will the clients be able to positively change, evolve, and heal from their habitual patterns.

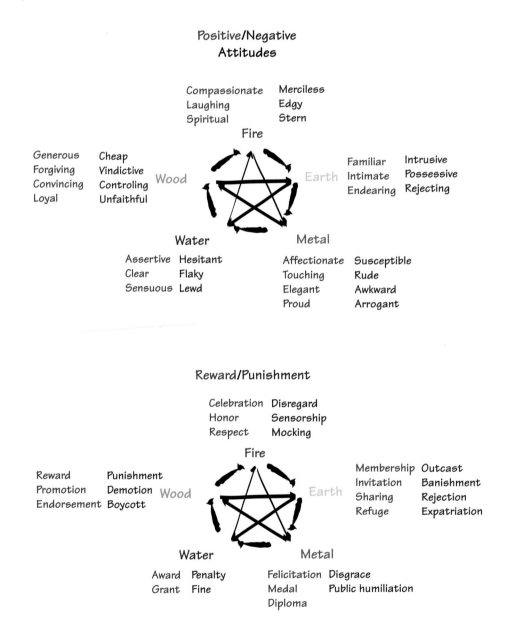

_____

Plate 22: Taoist perspective on attitudes and reactions—positive and negative attitudes, reward and punishment

Mental aspects, positive and negative emotions and the law of creation

Mental aspects and the law of creation

• Creativity and vision in Water bring intelligence in Wood.
• Intelligence and a clear mind in Wood feed a high spirit and wisdom in Fire.
• Wisdom in Fire is conducive to cleverness and practicality in Earth.
• Cleverness in Earth gives the mental perspective to allow emotional sensitivity and to validate feelings in Metal.
• Sensitivity and emotional maturity in Metal allow for inspiration and creative power in Water.

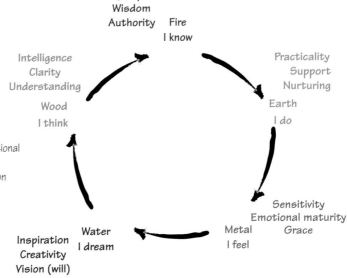

Positive emotions and the law of creation

• Gentleness in Water brings kindness and generosity in Wood.
• Generosity and kindness in Wood feed gratitude and enthusiasm in Fire.
• Joy and gratitude in Fire are conducive to satisfaction, inner peace, trust and trust in Earth.
• Trust and confidence in Earth develop honesty, pride and the courage to face emotions in Metal.
• Honesty and emotional maturity in Metal are conducive to calming and to the gentle power of sensuality in Water.

Negative emotions and the law of creation

• Fear in Water is conducive to anger in Wood.
• Anger and arrogance in Wood feed rage and hatred in Fire.
• Hatred and rage in Fire destabilize Earth and provoke anxiety and worry, preventing trust and confidence.
• Not trusting is detrimental to honesty and the sharpness of emotions in Metal: anxiety and lack of confidence in Earth feed sadness and depression in Metal.
• Dullness in Metal troubles Water: sadness and depression are conducive to fear of living and dullness of life.

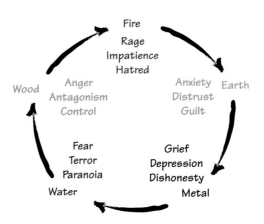

Plate 23: Mental aspects, positive and negative emotions, and the law of creation

How to use our positive mind to control negative feelings

There are 5 mental categories in Taoism. Thinking and intelligence are functions of the Wood elemental force. Other mental categories are spirit, wisdom and intuition in Fire, cleverness, practicality and harmonizing in Earth, sensitivity and honesty in Metal, and abstraction and creativity in Water.

For extraordinary results, to promote healing and life enjoyment, we need to use the positive aspects to neutralize the negative.
• Expanding feelings and sensitivity neutralizes anger.
• Clear, rational thinking stops anxiety.
• Practicality, cleverness, and stability of mind controls fear.
• Creativity makes rage disappear.
• With spirituality and love, depression vanishes.

When using the control cycle to transform negative feelings, remember that the Earth Force also exists in between all other elemental forces. So a transition time into any Earth attributes such as sensibility, comfort, nurturing and practicality might be necessary to prevent resistance to change.

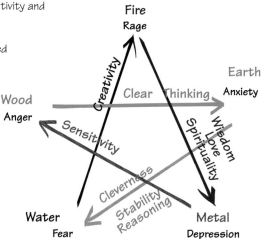

Ordinary, non-evolved way to deal with negative feelings

Ordinarily, because we are caught up in negativity, we react instinctively or we try to control negative feelings with another negativity such as controlling rage (Fire) with fear (Water), fear with blame and prejudice (Earth), anxiety (Earth) with aggressiveness (Wood), anger (Wood) with hopelessness (Metal), and depression (Metal) with impatience (Fire).

Plate 24: Control of negative feelings

Treating the pattern of fear

Fear can be viewed as Water rising out of control. Like a flood, fear is invading the system. It is necessary to consolidate the Earth so that it can contain the flood. Consolidating the Earth consists of doing everything possible to develop the feelings of safety, trust, unconditional support, comfort, nurturing, and satisfaction.

If you have the pattern of fear, you should eat regularly, make your home comfortable, cook your meals yourself, do some gardening, and work at feeling satisfied at all levels of existence.

• Earth Relationship Chi-Kung several times daily, cooking, and getting into a craft of any kind, or gardening to develop a sense of practicality, to strengthen the Earth energy within and to control the flow of Water.

• If the state of fear is chronic and your career is in finance and commerce, it would be advisable to make a career move toward one of the earthy professions such as engineering, construction, or farming.

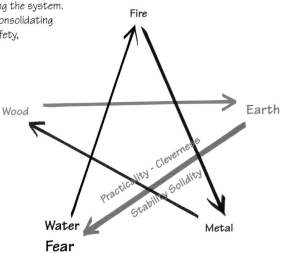

Plate 25: Treating the pattern of fear

Treating the pattern of anger

Anger is Wood, and therefore, can only grow and grow. Anger is a Yang emotion, very hot, consistent, superficial and powerful. It is at the surface of things and generally protects us from more deeply-seated negative feelings such as sadness, grief, fear, and terror that can rob us of our power. Anger is then an emotion that needs to be treated with respect because it is the ultimate protection against depression.

To outgrow anger, in Taoist terms, we need to "sharpen and polish our sword." This consists of breathing more fully and getting in touch with feelings and emotions. It takes strength to be sensitive.

• Breathing Chi-Kung daily, listening to music, and even studying music, and learning to play an instrument to appreciate it even more. Also spending more time on personal grooming, or getting into design, home decor, antiques, and spending more time refining yourself.

• If you have a chronic state of anger, and are in a Wood profession such as a legal, political or civic profession, military, or law enforcement it is advisable to make a change of profession toward Metal activities such as advertising, design, fashion, and landscaping.

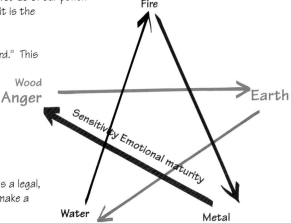

Plate 26: Treating the pattern of anger

Treating the pattern of impatience

Impatience kills. Every day many of us fall victim to accidents, heart attacks, and strokes as a result of having too much pressure in our heart. Pressure in the heart pushes us into being impatient to the point of sometimes being cruel and heartless. We then drive too fast, we stop trusting the process, and get into trouble by taking things into our own hands when things are going "too slow for us".

The heat is too high in our Inner Fire so we need to temper it with Water.

To empower our Water elemental force, we first need to sleep! Many impatient people are also insomniacs. When dominated by impatience, we need to invest in sleep, in abstraction, and the power of dreams.

• The Bone Breathing and Bone Dreaming meditations, swimming leisurely, vacationing and traveling, drawing or painting, sculpting, film or photography are good ways to progressively raise your Inner Water and effortlessly extinguish your excess Fire.

• If you have regular fits of rage, give up teaching and preaching (Fire) for a while and practice your Water Chi-Kung and figurative arts until you are able to do the most tedious kind of work without any feeling of impatience.

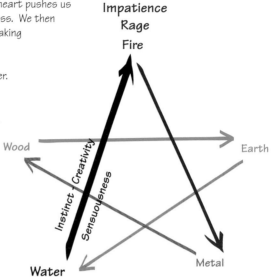

Plate 27: Treating the pattern of impatience

Treating the pattern of anxiety

Anxiety is Earth being destabilized. Once we feel anxious, we tend to look for external reasons for this and, of course, we find many. There is a strong irrational component to anxiety. We actually become prone to anxiety anytime things are not comfortable in our house or at work, and anytime we lose the rhythm of life, anytime we become irregular in our meals and sleep.

When our Earth is so destabilized, we need to strengthen our Inner Wood. Like working on a garden, weeding, watering and feeding it with regularity, we need discipline to help us find our rhythm, our comfort, and a sense of satisfaction.

• Study, learn a new skill or perfecting an old one. Invest in your education and self-development.

• Develop a project, an activity or business that can be shared with others.

• Practice relaxation, meditation, yoga, a martial art, dance, or Chi-Kung.

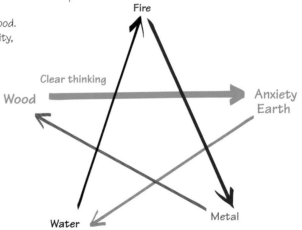

Plate 28: Treating the pattern of anxiety

Treating the pattern of depression

Depression is debilitating. Depression is about having lost enthusiasm for life. When we are depressed, we are constantly sending an inner message that says that since we are not enjoying life, we don't deserve to live.

Often, when depressed, we don't let ourselves know this and we pretend that we are actually doing fine because we are very busy. We actually have a tendency to do so much that we don't have time to stop and feel. This translates into workaholism, or a constant need for entertainment or activity. We then involve ourselves superficially into several unfulfilling activities instead of involving ourselves deeply into a fulfilling one.

We need to rekindle our Inner Fire, our spirit and passion.

• Deepen relationships that you feel you can put your enthusiasm into: friendships, parental, romance, pets, nature.

• Cultivate your spirit with humor and laughter.

• Enhance your spiritual practice with something new.

• Pay attention to what lights up your enthusiasm for life and go in that direction.

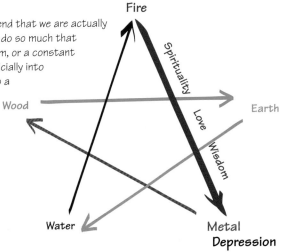

Plate 29: Treating the pattern of depression

Arts **and** Professions

Fire
Performing arts and show business: Theatre, opera, circus
Motion picture art
Comedy

Philosophy, religion, and spirituality
Health, healing, and medecine
Teaching and mastering of arts

Wood
Litterary arts: Writing, poetry, composition
Martial arts
Chi-Kung
Tai-Chi
Yoga
Sports

Management
Administration
Politics
Civil, legal, and military services
Law enforcement
Consulting
Education
Science
Research and development
Coaching and training

Earth
Craft-making: Ceramics, basketry, sewing, knitting, crocheting
Culinary arts
Gardening

Horticulture, farming
Engineering
Architecture
Construction
Carpentry, cabinetmaking
House-keeping
Restaurant and hotel industry

Water
Figurative arts: Painting, drawing, sculpting, filming

Finance: Banking, investment, real estate
Retail
Travel and tourism

Metal
Music
Flower arranging (Ikebana)
Tea ceremony (Cha Do)

Fashion and cosmetic industry
Perfumes, tailoring
Design: Automobile, furniture, Interior decorating, landscaping
Antique dealing
Advertisement
Public relations

Plate 30: Arts and professions

Healing through evolution

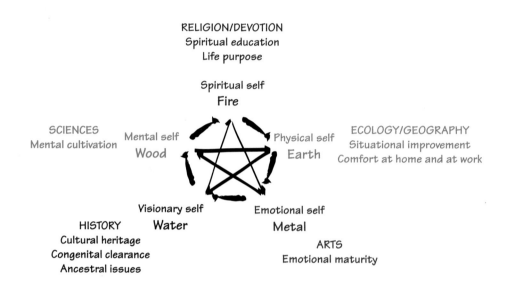

5 levels of cultivation:

• By refining ourselves through arts (Metal), we promote our emotional sensitivity and our ability to emotionally evolve (Water), and we have better control over our mental limitations (Wood).

• By studying our genealogy (Water), the evolution of humanity, its history, economy, and politics, it helps us understand (Wood) our parents and ancestors, and we get better control over our own life purpose, and spiritual life (Fire).

• By cultivating our mind, our ability to think clearly and develop understanding in life (Wood), we develop wisdom and rekindle our spirit (Fire) and we can improve our present life and situational environment (Earth).

• By practicing spirituality (Fire), we automatically improve our state of being (Earth) and get a better handle on our emotional life (Metal).

• By improving our situational environment (Earth), we facilitate our ability to mature emotionally (Metal), and we can have better control over our instinct, our congenital patterns of habits (Water).

Plate 31: Healing through evolution

CHAPTER ☆ 3

The Universal Laws of Life

The Taoist Alchemical System of the Five Elemental Forces

As mentioned in the preceding chapter, within our breath (the Metal elemental force) reside the mysteries of the alchemical principles of life. We understand the chemistry of breath, the chemical composition of the air we breathe, and the red blood cells that transport oxygen to every cell in our bodies. We understand the metabolic process of our bodies that mixes oxygen and energy from the food we eat and fires that spark of life in every cell. This is chemistry, or the composition of life. But what allows the chemistry of breath to happen? What is the principle that coordinates the entire body, regulating and extending the flow of life from every cell to our fingertips and beyond? That is alchemy, the principle that gives life to all the chemical components of a body and all their processes. Alchemy is what makes and keeps our metabolism alive.

We are familiar with the periodic table of the known chemical elements. We also know the five fundamental forces of physics that set the world in motion: the force of gravity, the centrifugal force, the magnetic force, and the weak and strong nuclear forces. Very little is known, however, of the alchemical forces of nature that allow life to happen. The ancient Taoist texts describe them as the "Five Elements," the "Five Phases," or the "Five Elemental Forces." These are the five natural principles activating life in the universe: the principle of Water, the principle of Wood, the principle of Fire, the principle of Earth, and the principle of Metal. Unlike their inanimate physical counterparts, the alchemical principles of the elemental forces of nature contain information and meaning so that, when they are working together harmoniously, they give life to our existence.

It is important to understand the Five Elemental Forces not as chemical elements, but as universal powers governed by their broad symbolic and alchemical meanings rather than by the narrow-viewed and reductionistic periodic table. Both have their applications for understanding our world, but remember that here we are studying health, life, and healing in the broadest sense possible.

Thus, *elemental Water* is not only the water present in the rivers, lakes, and oceans, or the water that runs in our sink, or the water contained in our bodies. It is the very principle of water, the spirit of water, the water of life. Elemental Water gives water its fluidity, its ability to evaporate, to crystallize when frozen, to sink without being forced, to naturally follow the path of least resistance, and yet be able to spring forth and gush out with tremendous power. Elemental Water also has cleansing and regenerative power and life-giving force. Water is the power of gentleness. In our bodies, Water manifests especially in our DNA, our genetic makeup that brings forth each generation. A healthy Water Chi—Chi being both energy and the information contained in it—manifests in our ability to be creative, prolific, progressive, innovative, adventurous, and determined. Within elemental Water reside our life force and willpower.

Elemental Wood is what makes life grow, develop, and multiply. Wood is the force that moves the sap in trees and makes plants grow. Wood Chi gives us our sexual drive and our ability to reach out, to play, to establish rules, to trade and exchange. In our bodies, a healthy Wood Chi manifests in our nervous system and in our ability to think clearly, make plans, theorize, cultivate ourselves, grow and prosper, be kind and generous, understand better and more clearly, and solve problems. Within elemental Wood is our intelligence.

Elemental Fire gives light and warmth to the universe. Fire is the power of high spirit, warmth, meaningful communication, love, passion, and enthusiasm, all of which reside in our heart and circulate in our blood. Elemental Fire manifests in our endocrine system and is responsible for the accuracy of communication, making sure that every single part of us knows what the other parts are doing. By extension, elemental Fire is responsible for our good internal communication and good communication within families, communities, and nations. A healthy Fire Chi provides meaningful communication, high spirit, joy, warmth, peace, love, respect, sacredness, purpose, and guidance in life. Within elemental Fire we find our spirit.

Elemental Earth contains everything related to unconditional support, nurturing, mothering, and comfort. Earth is the force of solidity, regularity, consistency, and balance that harmonizes all life functions in the universe. Elemental Earth is present in our digestive system and manifests in our muscles and our ability to move and act spontaneously, comfortably, and harmoniously in the present moment. The elemental force of Earth gives us the capacity to be and feel at the right place, at the right time, doing the right thing. A healthy Earth Chi gives us the ability to feel at home, to be comfortable, hospitable, nurturing, supportive, and conciliatory. It gives us a clear perspective, good judgment, sound practicality, and solid stability of mind and spirit. Within elemental Earth reside our sense of identity and authenticity.

Elemental Metal is the most abstract power in life. It rules feelings at both the physical and emotional levels. It directs our breath and is the surface tension between the different levels of existence and consciousness. Metal is the membrane, the inner bridge between wakefulness and dream, rational thinking and abstraction, literature and music, life and death. Breathing, from an alchemical perspective, and seen through the eyes of our Taoist ancestors, is a function of our inner Metal elemental force. Indeed, our lungs work exactly the way we use forks and knives to eat. Breathing is the ability to "cut" through the air and take only the oxygen. It is a marvelous feat that allows life-giving oxygen to be transported by the iron molecules in our red blood cells, energizing our whole metabolism. Similarly, Metal cuts through our life experience and allows us to absorb only what we can digest. Within elemental Metal resides our soul.

Once the Five Elemental Forces meet and interact harmoniously according to the laws of Tai-Chi, we have life.

The Law of Creation of the Elements of Life

Creation follows a natural order (see Plate 6). Starting from extreme Yin (the origin of things, the deepest, most hidden, most essential), Water, we have the following cycle:

- Water feeds Wood, or Wood takes its energy from Water.
- Then Wood fuels Fire, or Fire takes its energy from Wood.
- From Fire, we get ashes, the very nature of Earth, or Earth takes its energy from Fire.
- Within Earth grow minerals such as metal ore. We say, then, that Metal takes its energy from Earth. And Water is found deep inside Earth, and fluidity is the quality of the mineral found the deepest (extreme Yin) within the Earth (iron in its molten form).
- So, we say that Metal nourishes Water, and Water takes its energy from Metal.

Now, the law of creation is not enough to sustain itself. This one law alone would last no more than one cycle before everything disappeared in one chain reaction—all the Earth would condense into Metal, which would condense further into Water. Water would turn into Wood, all the Wood would burn in Fire … and nothing would be left! So there also has to be a law of control, which I call the law of preservation of the elements (see Plate 7).

The Law of Control and Preservation of the Elements of Life

Starting from Water again, we have a cycle that expresses the law of control and preservation of the elemental forces:

- Water creates Wood and Wood turns into Fire. To save some Wood from being completely consumed, Water has to control Fire.
- Wood fuels Fire and Fire gives rise to Earth in the form of ashes. Wood has to control Earth to protect the integrity of Fire.

- Fire turns into Earth and Earth into Metal. Fire has to control Metal to save Earth from being completely turned into Metal.
- Earth feeds Metal and Metal feeds Water. Earth has to control Water to preserve Metal.
- Metal nurtures Water and Water supports Wood. Metal has to cut Wood in order to conserve Water.

Now, this order requires some *imbalance* in order to have *real life,* rather than some perfect, well-ordered picture from a human demiurgic fantasy, where everything is in perfect balance, perfectly clean, and perfectly unreal. The world operates harmoniously in accordance with proportions, which are given to nature by Wu-Chi, in charge of measures and ratio in our world of Tai-Chi. Disproportion itself rarely gets to the point of chaos and complete destruction. Chaos itself has an order, such as the exquisitely precise ecological order of the tropical rain forest we call the jungle. That is, it has the ability to grow the maximum number of living organisms in the minimum amount of space.

The Law of Overpowering and Surrendering

Sometimes Water can be insufficient to douse a fire that's too big. Sometimes impatience and rage (Fire) are so strong that they overcome any kind of fear (Water). These are functions of the law of overpowering and surrendering (see Plate 8).

Metal can resist a Fire that is too weak. When the spirit (Fire) is very low, we can easily become upset or grief-stricken and succumb to depression (Metal).

The switchblade of a pocket knife (Metal) will break if we attempt to chop down a big tree (Wood) with it. When the rational mind is very well trained (Wood), it usually creates an escape or an armor against emotional sensitivity (Metal).

An unstable ground (Earth) prevents plants from taking root (Wood) and from growing. Similarly, a lack of good judgment and perspective (Earth) confuses rational thinking (Wood).

Excess Water can flood Earth. When experiencing great fright (Water), we may lose any common sense (Earth).

CHAPTER ☆ 4

The Daily Biological Clock and Human Behavior

The Meridian System

Color plates 9, 10, 11, 12, and 13 illustrate the points made in this chapter.

The meridian system is at the foundation of traditional Taoist medicine. Charts depicting the flow of energy in the body have been found not only in ancient China, the birthplace of Taoism, but also in India, Thailand, Indonesia, Japan, Tibet, and Nepal, with influences of energy flow being evident as far back as ancient Egypt. Even though the energy flow varies according to different schools of Traditional Chinese Medicine, throughout the ages, the principles and the general idea behind the meridian system have remained the same: Life force circulates in our bodies to all our internal organs through channels along our system of connective tissues, fasciae. This flow of energy and information, Chi, gives us our health, our morphology, our structural alignment, and is even responsible for our psychological profile and our emotional patterns.

Many Taoist monks and mystics, the scientists of those ancient times, noticed that particular parts of their bodies were systematically affected when their internal health was affected. For example, they realized that taking a walk after a meal helped their digestion and improved their mental acuity. This is because the Stomach and Spleen-Pancreas meridians, in charge of digestion, and the Liver and Gallbladder meridians, which control the nervous system and the brain, run through the legs. Low energy and old age are also felt through the legs because the Kidney and Bladder meridians, which hold vital force, also run in the legs. Arm and hand movements express our ability to trade and exchange, our communication skills, and manifest in our conversations and our ability to reach out and be in touch with our physical and social environment. This is because our Heart meridian, which reflects our inner Fire and our passions, our Heart Controller meridian, in charge of our endocrine system and our communication skills, and our Lung meridian, in control of our emotional life, are located in the arms and hands.

Still widely used today, the Traditional Chinese Medicine approach defines the most evolved and precise meridian system in existence. This meridian system is used in the meditation at the end of this chapter.

Plates 9 and 10 outline the twenty-four-hour biological clock and the structure of the meridian system. We are all part of nature and our lives follow the cyclical rhythms of the universe: the cycle of day and night, the cycle of seasons, the periodic cycle of lunar phases and ocean tides.

Thousands of years ago, our Chinese forefathers in Chi-Kung and Taoist yoga became aware of correlations among the diurnal phases, the physical and emotional needs of the body, and its corresponding flows of energy. They began to chart these correlations. They discovered periodic fluctuations of a "fluid," an inner flow, which are precisely governed by the movement of the sun rather than of the moon. They also noticed that their moods and physical needs changed regularly every two hours or so, consistently every day, regardless of the season or geographical location. In addition, certain parts of their body were energized, while other parts were at rest. Thus came the discovery of the fluctuations of the Chi flow within the acupuncture meridian system.

They also observed that the most severe breathing problems would appear around 3:00 in the morning, as did the most severe cases of nightmares. However, by 5:00 a.m., dreams would improve and bowel movements would be very satisfying. They then established that the hours between 3:00 a.m. and 7:00 a.m. would mark the high tide of energy for the power of Metal, the alchemical force that rules breath and elimination. Thus the peak of energy in the Yin Metal organ meridian or Lung meridian, is between 3:00 a.m. and 5:00 a.m., and the peak of energy in the Yang Metal organ meridian, also called the Large Intestine meridian, is between 5:00 a.m. and 7:00 a.m. Not having a bowel movement early in the morning sets us up for constipation.

After the first bowel movement upon arising, the next physical need is for food. Not just any kind of food, however, and not necessarily a big meal, and not always eaten in the company of others. We all have specific needs for breakfast, specific habits that aren't easily changed. Breakfast is a matter of preference, corresponding to the need for personal nurturing that requires satisfaction and establishes the quality of appetite for the rest of the day. Have you ever noticed that if you eat a very small meal or skip breakfast altogether, you won't be hungry for the rest of the day, or you will have poor digestion? But if you have a big satisfying breakfast, you will be hungry for lunch just a few hours later, and most likely, you will be able to enjoy a nice dinner early in the evening without experiencing any feeling of excess or digestive problems. So, the early Taoists decided that the hours between 7:00 a.m. and 11:00 a.m., which set the appetite and the rhythm of digestion for the whole day, would belong to the Earth elemental force, with its supportive attributes of balance, comfort, consistency, harmony, nurturing, satisfaction, and solidity. The hours of the Yang Earth organ meridian, also called the Stomach meridian, are between 7:00 a.m. and 9:00 a.m., and the hours of the Yin Earth organ meridian, or Spleen-Pancreas meridian, are between 9:00 a.m. and 11:00 a.m.

At the end of the morning, it is time for a mid-day break, time for socializing and eating lunch in the company of others. We are willing to make some concessions with the food as long as the company is good and the atmosphere light-hearted. This is the time for sharing a meal—high noon, the time of Cardiovascular Fire, where the spirit soars. It is a good time to exchange pleasantries over a hearty meal, as well as a good time to spend with family and friends. Our Taoist forefathers established that this would be the time of the Yin Cardiovascular Fire meridian, or Heart meridian, between 11:00 a.m. and 1:00 p.m., and the time of assimilation and digestion, with the Yang Cardiovascular Fire meridian, or Small Intestine meridian, between 1:00 p.m. and 3:00 p.m.

Next comes a very important time where our personal reaction is going to determine not only the quality of the rest of the day, but also of that evening. At the beginning of the afternoon, many of us become tired, so this is naturally a time to break for either a siesta, or for tea or coffee. It is actually the time to regenerate, the time of the Water elemental force. A nap taken during the afternoon will refresh our life force because this is the refreshing time of Water, with the Yang Water meridian, or Bladder meridian, between 3:00 p.m. and 5:00 p.m., and the Yin Water meridian, or Kidney meridian, between 5:00 p.m. and 7:00 p.m. Water is life. If life is not too stressful, such as when we are vacationing by the sea in a warm climate, and we need an extra boost to walk to a nearby beach, and have a nap there, then coffee is fine. However, if we need coffee in order to stay awake to meet a deadline at work, and we are under pressure, coffee will only cause problems by keeping us in the stress response and preventing us from resting even if we have the opportunity to do so. Take the break, but not the coffee! It is indeed much healthier to have a short nap instead, or just some rest and quality quiet time. Exhaustion shows around 6:00 p.m. to 7:00 p.m. when we work too hard.

The next period of time is the most outgoing social time of the day, the precious happy hour of Endocrine Fire, the social fire of communication, between 7:00 p.m. and 9:00 p.m. for the Heart Controller meridian, also called the Yin Endocrine Fire meridian, and 9:00 p.m. and 11:00 p.m. for the Triple Heater, or Yang Endocrine Fire meridian. This is the time when we don't care what we eat as long as the company is pleasant. It is the time for candlelight, intimacy, and socializing. In fact, preparation of the meal should focus primarily on social interaction and enjoyment. Sophisticated dishes, rare wines, exquisite desserts, and fine liqueurs are for dinner that is to be shared in good company. If we are rested and our mind is clear, we can really enjoy ourselves and one another. If, however, the day has been long, and we had to have a coffee boost earlier, we now feel rather wound up and tired at the same time. Therefore, we might feel the need to self-medicate with drinking a little too much alcohol and smoking tobacco to achieve a more manageable pace. In this case, our social interactions might not be very authentic or favorable.

Soon 11:00 p.m. rolls around. This is the Yang Wood time of the Gallbladder meridian from 11:00 p.m. to 1:00 a.m., and the Yin Wood or Liver meridian time from 1:00 a.m. to 3:00 a.m., the peak time for our nervous system and mental activity. If we had a pleasant social time earlier, we'll fall asleep very content. If we had a little too much to drink, though, and we didn't have a satisfying social interaction, we'll be obsessing about it until 2:00 a.m.! If we are not in bed yet, this is the time when conversations turn into arguments, and mere thinking turns into obsession. This is Wood time—time for growth and creativity when we are well rested, and time for obsessions and phobias when our nervous system is overstimulated, and we are tired. The best works of literature and fine art, and any kinds of projects, musical compositions, and planning have probably been conceived during the Wood time between 11:00 p.m. and 3:00 a.m. So, too, were all works of art representing obsessions, morbid themes, violence, destruction, and doom a result of stress and mental exhaustion. If our mind is able to rest and recuperate by sleeping during Wood time, then everything settles down during the subsequent Metal time of dreams and abstraction (3:00 a.m. to 7:00 a.m.). Then, upon arising, we find it easy to make clear decisions about the project at hand, as this is Earth time (7:00 a.m. to 11:00 a.m.), when creativity manifests effortlessly and spontaneously.

This twenty-four-hour clock shows how the meridians connect with one another. Like the old vinyl records with several songs recorded on one uninterrupted groove, the meridians are linked to one another in three solid and symmetrical loops, one on each lateral side of the body (left and right). Each loop consists of four meridians: two pairs of Yin and Yang meridians going from head to feet and from feet to chest, and from chest to hand and from hand to head.

To be more precise, the Stomach meridian from head to feet (Yang Earth, 7:00 a.m. to 9:00 a.m.) runs down each side of the front of the body (left and right) and down each leg to the feet where it connects to the Spleen-Pancreas meridian from feet to chest (Yin Earth, 9:00 a.m. to 11:00 a.m.) at the big toes, going up to the chest to connect to the Heart meridian from chest to hands (Yin Cardiovascular Fire, 11 a.m. to 1:00 p.m.), ending at the little fingers, connecting with the Small Intestine meridian from hands to head (Yang Cardiovascular Fire, 1:00 p.m. to 3:00 p.m.), and going to the sides of the face. This is the first loop of the meridian system, the *daytime loop* (see Plate 12).

Then the meridian system continues from the face into the Urinary Bladder meridian from head to feet (Yang Water, 3:00 p.m. to 5:00 p.m.), going down the back of the head and back of the body to the little toes to connect to the Kidney meridian from feet to chest (Yin Water, 5:00 p.m. to 7:00 p.m.), starting at the bottom of the feet and running up the very inside of the legs to the base of the collarbones in the chest. There it becomes the Heart Controller meridian from chest to hands (Yin Endocrine Fire, 7:00 p.m. to 9:00 p.m.), running down the arms to the middle fingers, and turns into the Triple Heater meridian from hands to head (Yang Endocrine Fire, 9:00 p.m. to 11:00 p.m.), which runs from the back of the ring fingers up to the sides of the head, encircling the ears where it connects to the Gallbladder meridian. This ends the second loop of the meridian system, the *evening loop* (see Plate 13).

From the head the meridian system becomes the Gallbladder meridian from head to feet (Yang Wood, 11:00 p.m. to 1:00 a.m.), running from the cranium down both sides of the body to the fourth toes, and coming back up the inside of the legs as the Liver meridian from feet to chest (Yin Wood, 1:00 a.m. to 3:00 a.m.), from the big toes to the chest where it connects to the Lung meridian. The Lung meridian from chest to hands (Yin Metal, 3:00 a.m. to 5:00 a.m.) runs along the arms to the thumbs, connects to the Large Intestine meridian from hands to head (Yang Metal, 5:00 a.m. to 7:00 a.m.), coming from the index fingers and going to the sides of the nose where it connects to the Stomach meridian. This completes the third loop of the meridian system, the *nighttime loop* (see Plate 13), and the process starts over for the next day.

Now that you are familiar with the meridian system and your biological clock, it is important to be in touch with it and to learn to respect its internal rhythm. Once you know your rhythm, you'll be able to play with it and compensate for excesses or deficiencies without running the risk of getting sick. For example, you might need to meet a deadline for an important project. Knowing your internal rhythm will allow you to know when to work and when to rest for optimum efficiency without the need for artificial stimulants with their negative side effects. Or perhaps you wish to celebrate and participate in sharing meals, wines, and activities that might be enjoyable, but that might not agree with your digestive system. Being in touch with your internal rhythm and body's reactions, you will be able to pace yourself and to combine food and drink, activities, and resting times, in a manner that supports and stimulates your system and prevents you from getting sick.

My old master use to say, "For good health and longevity, everything in moderation, including moderation!" Indeed, in order to enjoy life to its fullest, we never want to exceed in moderation! Doing your practice regularly, you will be able to strengthen and cleanse your body well enough to endure occasional excesses, which, of course, you will be able to fully enjoy without remorse.

Knowing your meridian system and the direction of its flow, you'll be able to make yourself healthier by using the power of your mind. Use the meridian charts at first to learn to guide your energy in your different body systems and to increase your intuition about yourself. Soon you will no longer need the charts because you will be able to feel your own meridians. With regular practice, you might even be able to feel the fluctuations of your Chi, predict when you are starting to get sick, and be able to prevent and reverse illnesses.

The Healing Lights and Inner Smile Acu-Meditation

This meditation has the effect of a complete acupuncture treatment (and thus it is called an acu-meditation). When practiced regularly, it promotes good health, vitality, and longevity. It will also enhance your emotional maturity, stimulate your creativity, cultivate and open your mind, and raise your enthusiasm for life.

- Find a comfortable and peaceful place where you won't be disturbed for an hour or so. Tell people around you not to disturb you, and turn phone ringers and answering machines off, if you can.

- Sit comfortably with your back straight but not stiff. Feel free to move and adjust your body position to avoid any discomfort. It is okay to sit in an armchair as long as your back is supported in an erect position. Put a step stool or a pillow under your feet so they are not dangling, or sit comfortably crossed-legged, Indian-style, or on your heels, Japanese-style.

- Breathe calmly and center your breath behind your navel, sending your in-breath to your pelvic floor and sacrum and letting it rise slowly up your back all the way inside your shoulder blades. Drop the weight of all your bones with each out-breath.

- Keep relaxing and calming your breath until it becomes easy and slow.

- Take the time to sink yourself into a comfortable inner smile bath, as if you were immersing yourself into a bathtub full of inner smiles. Let your body slowly soak up these inner smiles like a sponge (see *Healing from Within,* p. 273, on the inner smile bath).

- Feel the whole length of your meridian system smiling on both sides of your body at the same time: your Lung meridians from your chest to your thumbs, your Large Intestine meridians from your index fingers to the sides of your nose. Smile in your Stomach meridians from your cheeks down the front of your body to your second toes and up your Spleen-Pancreas meridians from your big toes to your chest. Smile in your Heart meridians from your chest to your little fingers and in your Small Intestine meridians from your little fingers to the sides of your face. Smile in your Bladder meridians from the inside corners of your eyes, up your head and down your back to your little toes, and in your Kidney meridians from the bottom of your feet, up the inside of your legs to your collarbones in your chest. Smile in your Heart Controller meridians from your chest to your middle fingers and in your Triple Heater meridians from your ring fingers to the sides of your head by your ears. Smile in your Gallbladder meridians from your head to your fourth toes and in your Liver meridians from your big toes to your chest.

- In front of you, at the level of your mid-eyebrow, visualize a bright purple star—very bright, very purple or violet, shining so brightly that it can be seen all the way from outer space.

- Feel this bright purple star charging up with the regenerative power of nature, the healing power of God, the healing power of all the saints and mystics, and all the spiritual masters that you know of and believe in.

- Draw that purple star to your mid-eyebrow until you feel some itchiness, some warmth, and your eyes feel like they are tearing.

- Go deep within your heart and gather all the feelings that nourish your spirit, everything that no one can take away from you: your beliefs, the things you like most in life, the people you love, your favorite animals, favorite trees, favorite stars, favorite music, favorite rhythm, favorite place on earth.

- Bring these feelings of love and passion to that purple light between your eyes, adding to the brightness and the feelings of warmth.

- Condense the purple light into a precious purple crystal made of absolute feelings of love and warmth. A purple or violet crystal, very shiny and bright, holding all the healing powers of creation.

- Feel and visualize that powerful violet crystal right between your eyes and let it shine there for a while. Feel your brain progressively charging up with mental power, a power of absolute focus and determination.

- Slowly and carefully, bring that shiny violet crystal from your mid-eyebrow to your heart, and see it turning bright red like a ruby in the sun, charging your heart with warmth, love, enthusiasm, and high spirit.

- Now, bring your crystal to your lower abdomen and see it turning deep and dark like a smoky quartz, or deep black like obsidian. Feel the power of that crystal charging you with creativity, willpower, life-giving force, and the power of all your unmanifested potential.

- Feel the power of focus and determination between your eyes with the bright purple crystal. Feel the power of love, high spirit, and enthusiasm in your heart with the bright red ruby. Feel the creative power in your lower abdomen with the deep black obsidian. Keep them there. Keep the awareness of their forces throughout this whole meditation.

- Be aware of the flow of life circulating in your body. Feel your blood circulating in your veins.

- Feel the general flow of your Yin meridian system flowing up the inside of your legs to your abdomen and to your internal organs, and from your internal organs out to your chest and down the inside of your arms to your hands.

- Feel the general flow of your Yang meridian system flowing from the back of your hands to your head and down your back, front, and sides to your feet.

- Be aware of the bright purple crystal between your eyes charged with the healing power of the universe. Direct that crystal inside your body's energetic system to revitalize it.

- Feel that crystal between your eyes, charging with the alchemical force of Wood—the principle of cultivation, of clarity and understanding; the principle of intelligence and problem solving; the principle of growth, production, planning, generosity, and abundance.

- Visualize that powerful crystal turning bright green inside your head like an emerald in the light.

- Feel that bright green crystal dividing into two and entering both of your eyes. Feel your eyes turning bright green, calming-but-invigorating green, very pleasant to the eyes.

- Feel and visualize the bright green light spreading to the optic nerves at the back of your eyes, and spread the bright green light to your brain.

- Feel the bright green light filling your brain with a soothing greenness, as if you were looking at a field of new grass in the spring sun—very green, very bright, but very calming.

- Feel the bright green light spreading to your spinal cord and to all the nerves in your body, all the way to the surface of your skin, to all your internal organs, and to every nerve plexus.

- Look inward at your liver and gallbladder under the right side of your rib cage and flash the bright green light at them. Take the time to see your whole liver turning green. If there are any dark spots in your liver, any places in your liver you have a hard time visualizing, keep flashing the bright green light there.

- Smile at your liver until you get a smile back.

- Feel your bright green crystals in your eyes charged with healing energy and, slowly and carefully, bring them to the outer corners of your eyes, to your Gallbladder meridians, your Yang Wood meridians.

- Slowly and systematically, move the bright green crystals along the Wood meridian system to clarify it, opening all obstructions, and moving all stagnation.

- Bring the bright green crystals along the Gallbladder meridians on both sides of your head to your temporal bones, encircling your ears and zigzagging up to your forehead and back to the base of your skull, down your neck to your seventh cervical vertebra, down the sides of your body and the sides of your legs to your fourth toes.

- In your feet, the bright green crystals travel to your big toes where they connect to the Yin Wood meridians, your Liver meridians.

- There, the bright green crystals travel up the inside of your legs, penetrate your sexual and reproductive organs, continue up your abdomen through your colon, penetrate the liver on your right side and your pancreas on your left side, cross your diaphragm, your chest, your throat, your jaws, and enter your eyes and brain.

- Bring the crystals back into your chest, in your lungs. There, they are going to turn bright and white like the reflected sunshine on fresh-fallen snow.

- Feel the bright white light emanating from the crystal as pure healing energy.

- Feel the bright white light shining from both crystals, energizing and clarifying both lungs.

- Take the time to feel the coolness of the bright white light from both crystals penetrating the whole volume of your lungs, awakening the power of Metal with all its attributes of sharpness, smoothness, coolness, uprightness, righteousness, sensitivity, honesty, emotional maturity, and courage.

- Feel the power of the crystals and the bright white light clarifying your feelings, validating your deepest and most hidden emotions.

- Feel the bright white light and the healing power of your Metal elemental force spreading to your skin, enhancing your ability to "be in touch," to feel, to appreciate. Feel it through the whole length of your large intestine and through the whole volume of your lungs.

- Feel the crystals in the lungs rising in your chest and coming out near your shoulders at the Lung meridians, also called Yin Metal meridians, slowly and gently flowing down your arms to your thumbs. Make sure you can visualize the bright white light along the whole length of both of your Lung meridians.

- Feel and visualize the crystal and the bright white light moving from your thumbs to your index fingers, entering your Large Intestine meridians, or Yang Metal meridians.

- Visualize the bright white light flowing up your arms all the way to your seventh cervical vertebra, then along your shoulders, up your neck, and crossing each other under your nose at the side of the base of your nose.

- Now, bring both crystals from both sides of your nose to your cheeks. There, the crystals turn golden as they enter the Stomach meridians, or Yang Earth meridians, and flow around the jaws and down your neck to your chest, crossing both nipples, and down your abdomen and the middle of both legs, the middle of both ankles, to your second toes.

- There, your bright golden crystals enter the Spleen-Pancreas meridians on the outside of your big toes, also called Yin Earth meridians, and flow up the inside of your legs to your abdomen where they enter the digestive organs. There, they harmonize the digestive functions and provide all the attributes of Earth energy: nurturing, satisfaction, contentment, unconditional support, solidity, consistency, balance, harmony, regularity, comfort, practicality, and good judgment.

- Feel these Earth qualities being carried through the golden light and feeding all the muscles in your body with a sense of satisfaction, relaxation, and peace.

- Visualize and feel both crystals in your body moving from the digestive system to your chest, where they turn bright red as they enter your heart, your Yin Fire organ, and radiate beautiful love energy, stimulating your spirit, soothing any scars you have there with the warm feeling of a magic balm.

- Bring the bright red light from your heart to your tongue, and to your eyes. There is a direct connection there, very easy to find—a connection that doesn't tolerate lies or even bad language. A connection that establishes the interrelationship between your spoken words and your spirit. A connection that makes you speak from your heart and nourishes your spirit instead of destroying it. Let the Fire energy penetrate your tongue and burn warm and clean, without smoke, in both your heart and your tongue together, nourishing the principles of high-level communication, high spirit and joy, intuition, consciousness, truthfulness, conscience, respect, and sacredness.

- Bring the bright red light in your abdomen inside your small intestine, your Yang Fire organ, where your spirit manifests, where your gut feelings originate. This is where you have the sense of being on the right track, the place within you where you get the sense of true, genuine, and spontaneous laughter.

- Smile at your small intestine. Breathe into it, listen to it, feel the warmth in it.

- Bring the bright red light and the warmth of your spirit to your blood and feel every blood cell in your body warm, happy, and smiling.

- Bring your bright red crystals from your heart to your Heart meridians, your Yin Fire meridians, under your arms. Then, bring the bright red crystals down the inside of your arms to your little fingers, where they connect to your Yang Fire meridians, your Small Intestine meridians. From there, they go up the back of your arms, across your shoulder blades to your seventh cervical vertebra, and up your neck to the sides of your face.

- From the sides of your face, your bright red crystals cross to the other side of the eyes near your nose at the tear ducts, the first points of your Bladder meridians, or Yang Water meridians.

- There, your crystals turn deep blue—very deep, very blue like the ocean. From there, your deep blue crystals go up your forehead and flow down the back of your head, the back of your neck, down your back like a soft shower all the way to your feet, to your little toes. There, they connect to your Yin Water meridians, your Kidney meridians, at the Bubbling Spring at the bottom of your feet, your ground-wire connection with the earth.

- There, you are going to feel the genuine power of Water. Very strong, but extremely gentle—the power of gentleness, the power of sinking effortlessly following the path of least resistance, with the ability to spring forth with tremendous power. Water is the power of cleanliness, clarity, fluidity, and freshness; it is the power of regeneration, creativity, will, and life-giving force.

- Feel and visualize your deep blue crystals entering the Yin Water meridians, or Kidney meridians, from under your feet, going up the inside of your legs to your sacrum and your abdomen, all the way up to your collarbones.

- From your sacrum, visualize the deep blue light entering your spine and flowing to all your bones, to your kidneys, and your ears.

- Visualize the crystals in your chest now turning purple, reflecting a beautiful violet light and entering your Yin Endocrine Fire meridians, or Heart Controller meridians, and going down the middle of the inside of your arms to your middle fingers, where they enter your Triple Burner meridians, your Yang Endocrine Fire meridians, in your ring fingers. From there, they continue up the middle of the back of your arms and meet at your seventh cervical vertebra, then go up to the sides of your head by your ears, your temporal bones, your eyebrows, and meet again between your eyebrows, where they inwardly connect with your chain of main endocrine glands. (The energetic centers corresponding to these physical endocrine centers are the Chakras.)

- Take the time to energize each main endocrine gland and reinforce its connection within the network of communication.

- Picture and feel your pineal and pituitary glands shining extremely brightly between your eyes like beautiful twin violet stars shining so brightly that they can be seen all the way from outer space.

- Bring the violet light to your throat, and feel your thyroid center there being activated and shining very brightly.

- Bring the same bright violet light to your thymus in your chest above your heart, and feel it charged and shining very brightly.

- Feel and visualize the same bright violet light in your solar plexus, shining the energy of your pancreas there.

- Bring that same violet light to your "Door of Life," that place in your lower back opposite your navel, and feel the energy of your adrenals being gathered there and brightly shining that violet light.

- Feel and visualize the same bright violet light energizing your reproductive glands in your lower abdomen—ovaries for women and testicles for men—and let the bright violet light shine from your pelvic floor.

- Feel and visualize the seven main endocrine centers in your body shining that same violet light very brightly, shining together like a very bright constellation.

- Visualize the healing power of that violet light in a beautiful smile—an irresistible and genuine smile like a baby's smile, a beautiful woman's smile, a saint's smile—making that bright purple constellation not only very bright, but also very warm and balmy.

- Let the violet light travel back and forth to all the stars of your endocrine glands, energizing them, balancing them, with each one covering for the others in case any are weak or have been surgically removed.

- Take the time to feel and visualize your whole meridian system with all its internal connections to your internal organs, all the different colors flowing very smoothly and brightly.

- Feel the circulation of the Chi and the different lights in your meridian system—up your Yin meridians on the inside of your legs, the front of your torso, inside your arms to your hands, and inside your Yang meridians from the back of your arms to your head and down your back, sides, and front of your body and your legs.

- Keep the feelings and the memory of this practice deep within you.

CHAPTER ★ 5

The Seven Informational Levels of the Small Heavenly Cycle

The Seven Steps of Individuation of the Microcosmic Orbit

The Small Heavenly Cycle, also known as the Microcosmic Orbit, is the legendary practice that leads to the opening of the "third eye" and enlightenment—the ability to see clearly, perceive reality, be authentic, and be completely human.

The Small Heavenly Cycle is composed primarily of seven levels, which correspond to seven levels of individuation and consciousness. These seven levels need to be cleared of parasitic emotional charges in order to allow a healthy flow of life force and the attainment of true humanity. At the energetic level, this means attainment of a solid anchoring in pragmatic reality while being open to the marriage of heaven and earth and the fulfillment of our destiny.

The first level contains the sexual center from which energy is created for the enjoyment of life. It contains three centers:

- Starting from the ground level at the pelvic floor, we have the area related to comfort and rest, the ability to feel unconditionally supported and validated. When contracted or weak, this area of the body holds emotional charges preventing the full enjoyment of comfort. In this case, we might find it difficult to receive or give support or to feel free to be authentic. We can never feel at home. We can never really be ourselves, and we feel like we have to play a role in order to be accepted. Being comfortable here means that we can naturally enjoy our place in the sun. We enjoy the earth, and we feel like the earth is enjoying us. We trust the earth and existence to support us.

- The coccyx at the end of our sacrum is our tailbone. Even though we don't have a real tail, the energy there gives us momentum for life. A tucked-in coccyx is a sign of depression—people often get chronically depressed after a fall on their coccyx and any activity feels like a chore. At the other extreme, a chronically protruding sacrum and coccyx is often a sign of submission. An aligned coccyx, free of tension and stagnation, means that we can gather momentum and easily spring into action.

- The sexual center is the center of enjoyment. This does not mean that we have to have sex continually in order to enjoy life, but that any enjoyment involves the use of sexual energy. Sexual energy is the strongest energy we have. It is the power of life-giving force, creativity, willpower, determination—the power without which we wouldn't care about meeting anyone. Without it, we couldn't be social. We constantly use our sexual energy when we are creative, when we communicate, and for any type of relationship.

When working harmoniously together, these three centers form our first level of individuation: our ability to feel life and to enjoy it.

The second level of individuation represents our basic life force.

- On our back, opposite our navel, is the Door of Life, our lifetime "bank account" containing our genetic background and inheritance—our ancestral assets, birth gifts, karma. When we experience chronic pain here, we often have some ancestral issues concerning our inheritance. Maybe we inherited too many debts and unfinished business from our bloodline. We need to heal from the past and trade old values for new ones.

    When strong and relaxed here, we feel the gentle power of life running through our veins, and we can relax and accomplish anything without forcing.

- At our navel, we store our daily budget in life force currencies with energy immediately available for our activities and projects. This is the energetic hub of our body. Tension and imbalance here point to the different places in us that need attention.

Each level supports the next one. So, just as the enjoyment of life is the necessary support for our personal energy, this basic life force of our second level is necessary for the fulfillment of the *third level of individuation, self-consciousness.*

- On our back, right behind our solar plexus at the eleventh thoracic vertebra (T11), is the center that gives us choice. T11 is the vertebra that allows us to bend over and backward, rotate, and change direction. When stiff or painful here, we are confronted with emotions that keep us trapped and make us feel stuck. We need to be able to perceive the energetic chains that prevent us from being ourselves.

   When relaxed and free here, we can easily change direction to adapt to the evolution of life.

- Our solar plexus is probably the most emotionally susceptible place in our body. Here we hide all the emotional charges connected with how we are made to feel about ourselves, and all the emotions related to self-consciousness, shame, guilt, and poor self-esteem. When free of these emotional negativities, we know ourselves and have a strong sense of authenticity. We feel comfortable and at ease in any situation.

Only when we know ourselves can we manifest our spirit freely. *The fourth level of individuation relates to spirit and freedom.*

- On our back, opposite our heart, is the place of burden. This is where we carry our baggage, our unfinished business, our obligations and duties. When the load is too heavy, we cannot open our heart. When our heart is open, our spirit is free to be.

- Our heart center is where we carry our passions, our enthusiasm for life, our joys and spirit. This is where our wisdom, intuition, and conscience reside.

   When relaxed, this location lets us know our life purpose, what we like and don't like, who we are supposed to be with, where we are supposed to spend our life.

Once we are in touch with our spirit, we want to share it. This brings us to the *fifth level of individuation,* which is about communication.

- At the base of our neck, at the seventh cervical vertebra (C7), we have the center that allows us to reach out, to trade, to exchange, to give and receive. When burdened here, we feel like the weight of the whole world is upon our shoulders, and we are unable to ask for help.

  When free of tension here, we can easily open our arms to the world.

- Our throat is our center of expression and verbalization. It is also connected with our ability to swallow our emotions.

The next level of individuation, our *sixth level, is about introspection and consciousness.*

- At the base of our skull is our center of abstraction, where our dreams emerge. It encompasses the widest spectrum of consciousness and provides the mind with insight.

- At the mid-eyebrow, we have our center for clarity and understanding, logic, and rationality.

  When these centers are open and relaxed, we are clearly in touch with ourselves and others.

The *seventh level of individuation covers the full Heavenly Cycle within the limits of our physical body.* It connects the crown to the pelvic floor and aligns the seven levels at the Central Channel to form the chain of Chakras, the centers of energy and information manifested physiologically in our main endocrine glands: the pituitary and pineal in our head, the thyroid in our throat, the thymus in our chest, the pancreas at our solar plexus, the adrenals at the level of our navel, and our reproductive glands—ovaries for women and testes for men—in our lower abdomen.

- The top of our head, or crown, connects us with guidance and spiritual life.

  This is the place where we send our prayers and receive answers to our questions regarding our life.

By training to keep all these centers free of tension, we enhance our capacity to be truly human.

The Human Potential Enhancing Meditation:
Opening the Seven Loops of Individuation

First Loop:
Earth Foundations (Ground Level)—Cultivating Support, Comfort, and Enjoyment of Life

For the pelvic floor (perineum), sacrum, and sexual center:

- Initiate Earth Relationship Chi-Kung and be aware of the unconditional nature of the Earth support.

- Imagine that you have been walking for a long time, that you are very tired, and you are just sitting down. Be aware of your pelvic floor opening to the feeling of rest and comfort.

- Feel the Earth energy as the chair you are sitting on. Feel the same sense of rest and support in your feet, legs, hips, and pelvis, and relax into them.

- Take the time to really enjoy that moment, and be aware of how that feeling of relaxation and ease spreads throughout your body.

- Smile in your feet, in your legs, and pelvis, and be aware of the earth smiling back at you by making itself softer and more comfortable.

- Imagine now that you have been resting for a long time, and that you now feel like moving and doing something.

- Feel the Earth energy moving from your pelvic floor to your tailbone and sacrum, and feel the accumulation of momentum there. Feel like you are bending forward to get up and move.

- Feel the energy moving across to your sexual center, moving you in the direction of doing something enjoyable. The sexual direction is not only for sex, but for all sorts of enjoyment in general, and interrelationship in particular, regardless of sexual activities.

- Slowly, circulate the energy from your sexual center to your pelvic floor, emphasizing the need to balance activity with rest. Then move the energy from your pelvic floor to your sacrum, emphasizing the fluctuation between rest and momentum. Move the energy again from your sacrum to your sexual center, emphasizing the need to enjoy whatever activities you engage in.

- Slowly, alternate from one center to the other, paying attention to your inner feelings and listening to your inner voice.

- Let a sense of strength and solidity build in this first level of individuation. This is your base support, your foundation to your right to enjoy life like everything else alive on earth. You are alive, you made it! Life is already supporting you. Use that support!

When the energy flows freely in this level of our Microcosmic Orbit, we experience an unconditional trust in life and confidence in our destiny. We can enjoy life, and we naturally work to make life enjoyable for others and ourselves. We trust our support system, and we can be trusted to support others.

When the energy is restricted here, the tendency is not to trust anyone or anything, and to put safety before comfort. We trust people who make us feel safe rather than comfortable, and we are unable to feel support from our parents or friends, regardless of their reliability. Our fear prevents us from enjoying ourselves. There is no momentum in our life; everything seems to be static, and it takes a tremendous amount of effort to accomplish anything. Our support for others turns into a prison for them. We tend to protect them rather than accept and support them for who and what they are, in whatever direction they want to go.

Second Loop:
(Energetic and Informational Level)—Cultivating and Enriching Our Ancestral Inheritance

Being pulled by heavenly forces, our energy moves vertically from our feet, legs, hips, and pelvis to our lower back and abdomen—to our Door of Life, the zone of manifestation of the power of the Water elemental force and its life-giving information contained in our genes, and to our navel, the center of our bodies, the place where we originated and grew from embryo to fetus and became a human being, and from where we continue to grow as a human soul.

For the Door of Life, and our navel:

- Feel the energy circulating strongly in the first loop of your Microcosmic Orbit—pelvic floor, sacrum, and sexual center—firmly supported by the unconditional support and acceptance of the earth.

- Feel a gentle pull from the top and back of your head and let some of that energy from the first loop be pulled up your back to your Door of Life, on your back behind your navel, like a tide being pulled by the full moon.

- Let the strong wave of energy roll over from your back at your Door of Life to your front at your navel, and let the energy flow back down to your sexual center and your pelvic floor like a heavy wave. Pump it back up to your Door of Life and across to your navel in a continuous flow.

This is your second level of individuation, your personal energy center at your navel fed by your ancestral background, your biological inheritance and your genes, felt in the strength of your lower back and your kidneys.

When the energy flows freely in this level of our Microcosmic Orbit, we experience the strength of our genes. We experience calm and confidence. Our full life potential can be manifested in self-development and health.

When the energy is restricted here, we feel powerless, tired, and unable to manifest ourselves fully. Even though we are in constant need, we have difficulty appreciating the gifts that come our way, and it seems as though our needs become a bottomless pit from which no sense of satisfaction can emerge.

These first two loops are the lower part of the Microcosmic Orbit, the most fundamental part, the foundation of our consciousness. Everything alive has them. This is the cycle of life and marks the basic natural rights of everything alive: unconditional support and nourishment from earth, and guidance and inheritance from heaven in the form of the information contained in the genes. This is the basic joy we experience in life through enjoying our children and grandchildren, and it manifests in everything we create.

Third Loop:
(Physical Level)—Self-Awareness, Identity, and Authenticity

Once we have a strong foundation in the enjoyment of life and personal power, we can develop a strong sense of identity and a choice in our direction in life.

For T11, and our solar plexus:

- Feel the strong current of Chi circulating in the first two loops of your Microcosmic Orbit, with a strong sense of support and personal strength.

- Feel the upper pull of the heavenly force and draw some of that energy up your back to T11, the vertebra behind your solar plexus that bends and rotates more easily than the others.

- Feel your middle back releasing, opening to a sense of flexibility, adaptability, and change.

- Feel the Chi crossing over to your solar plexus, opening you to a sense of identity, your authentic sense of self.

- Feel the Chi flowing back down the front of your body to your navel, sexual center, and perineum, and being pumped up your back to your sacrum, Door of Life, T11, and crossing over to your solar plexus in a continuous flow.

When the energy flows freely in this level of our Microcosmic Orbit, we are flexible, tolerant, and able to see the big picture from a fair perspective. We have a sense of self-reliance, self-respect, and respect for the differences in others. We appreciate diversity and are adaptable, hospitable, congenial, and firm in our opinions, yet conciliatory. We enjoy making life comfortable for others and ourselves.

When the energy is restricted here, we can never feel satisfied. We lose our sense of self-respect and seek to conform to the standards of others, easily developing a chronic sense of anxiety, even panic, about others being "different" or about ourselves not "fitting in." Self-consciousness gets the better of us. Constantly worrying about what others think of us, we become self-centered and selfish.

Fourth Loop:
(Emotional Level)—Freedom of Spirit

A solid sense of identity provides support for our spirit.

For T4 (the freedom center), and the heart center:

- Pull a wave of Chi up your back to T4 behind your heart and allow that vertebra to release any burden as you develop a feeling of freedom to follow your destiny.

- Feel the Chi crossing over to your heart, opening the door to your spirit. Feel the Chi flowing down the front of your body to your solar plexus, navel, sexual center, and perineum, and springing up your back to your sacrum, Door of Life, T4, crossing over to your heart in a continuous flow.

When the energy flows freely in this level of our Microcosmic Orbit, we cannot lie. We have a sense of honesty and integrity. Freedom and the spirit of inquiry feel more important to us than innocence, ignorance, and the false security of denial.

When the energy is restricted here, we are unable to communicate meaningfully with others, or even with ourselves. We fall victim to hopelessness and are unable to love or feel loved.

Fifth Loop:
(Verbal Level)—Altruism, Communication, Reaching Out, Exchange

Once we find our spirit, we need to let it speak. The throat is the center of communication. Our seventh cervical vertebra, located at the base of our neck, is strategically placed between our shoulders. This is the starting point for our arms and hands, with our prehensile thumbs, which allow our unique mental coordination and intelligence. The throat center not only enables us to physically reach out toward others, to touch, move, and build things, but is also the place where we develop articulation of our thoughts.

For C7, and the throat:

- Pull a wave of Chi up your back to the base of your neck and loosen up there to allow the energy to flow down your arms, to your hands and fingers.

- Let the Chi from your C7 cross over to your throat and flow down the front of your body to your heart, solar plexus, navel, sexual center, and perineum, and up your back to your sacrum, Door of Life, T11, T4, C7, then crossing over to your throat, flowing down the front of your body and up your back again in a continuous wave.

When the energy flows freely in this level of our Microcosmic Orbit, we have an all-embracing sense of oneness and understanding at the physical, mental, emotional, and spiritual levels. We can reach out toward others and be very social. This is the center that allows us to give and receive, and to easily articulate and verbalize our thoughts and feelings.

When the energy is restricted here, we often hold a lot of tension in our neck and shoulders as if we were carrying the weight of the whole world. We feel overburdened and are unable to take in anything. (It is difficult to open our arms when carrying a big load on our shoulders!) This then makes it difficult to learn anything or to even reach out for help. We feel the burden of loneliness and isolation.

Sixth Loop:
(Mental Level)—Perception, Vision, Understanding

When we perfect our communication skills with others, we arrive at our next level of introspection. This level is directed by our level of abstraction and dreams situated at the base of our skull and by our mid-eyebrow, our center of clarity and understanding.

For the base of the skull (the Jade Pillow), and the mid-eyebrow (the third eye):

- Pull a wave of Chi up your back to the base of your skull.

- Let the Chi from the base of your skull cross over diagonally to your mid-eyebrow and flow down the front of your body to your throat, your heart, solar plexus, navel, sexual center, and perineum, and up your back to your sacrum, Door of Life, T11, T4, C7, and the base of your skull, then crossing over to your mid-eyebrow, and down the front of your body and up your back again in a continuous wave.

When the energy flows freely in this level of our Microcosmic Orbit, we are open-minded. Through our dreams or dreamlike states, we possess the vision and ability to perceive things, which our rational mind cannot analytically comprehend. From here, we develop our extrasensory capacities.

When the energy is restricted here, mental activity dulls, personality becomes identified with unrealistic images, and we can easily get lost mentally, seeking distraction through meaningless entertainment. Lacking vision and foresight, we then become narrow-minded and unable to learn. This sets us up to become easy victims of conditioning, propaganda, abusive advertisements, and illusions and delusions of all sorts.

Seventh Loop:
(Spiritual Level)—Transcendence and Convergence with Spirit, Guidance

With our lower six levels flowing smoothly and unimpeded, we now have clear communication between heaven and earth through the Central Channel. This is the level of complete listening and receptivity, the level of conception of life purpose and realization of free will (organizing ourselves according to our life purpose). This is the center of communication with the higher self and beyond, the level of convergence with Spirit or transcendence, the place where we send prayers and receive answers.

For the perineum, and crown of the head:

- Pull a wave of Chi up your back all the way to the top of your head.

- Open the top of your head and feel a direct connection with your pelvic floor through your Central Channel.

- Let the Chi flow from the top of your head down the front of your forehead to your mid-eyebrow and down the front of your body to your throat, heart, solar plexus, navel, sexual center, and perineum, and up your back to your sacrum, Door of Life, T11, T4, C7, the base of your skull, to the top of your head, to your mid-eyebrow, and flowing down the front of your body and up your back again in a continuous wave.

When the energy flows freely in this level of our Microcosmic Orbit, we feel guided by higher forces, which surpass human understanding.

When the energy is restricted here, we lose our sense of direction in life and might feel forsaken and purposeless.

Note to Practitioners: The flow of Chi in any of these energy centers can be restricted by emotional charges trapped in these areas. It is difficult to know which came first: the physical restriction or the psychological profile. My approach is to work with both aspects at the same time. I call this the *global body attitude* approach, by which I simultaneously treat the person from the internal and external structural perspectives, the metabolic aspects, and from the emotional places within them.

Opening the Microcosmic Orbit Meditation

- Find a comfortable sitting position where you can relax with your back straight but not stiff. Back supports are okay. Let your breathing slow down. Bring your awareness behind your navel and build an empty sphere there, letting that sphere expand during inhalation and shrink back during exhalation. Put your awareness on the quality of that sphere expanding and shrinking, on the rhythm of your breath, and keep it there while you do the Inner Smile meditation.

- Be aware of your perineum, or pelvic floor, and expand your breath there. Let your weight sink and build a feeling of comfort.

Feel the support of the earth through your "sit bones," your spine, and your whole body. Breathe in that sense of support and comfort. Connect in space and time with a place of absolute comfort, unconditionally supportive and nurturing for you. Relax in your sitting position and feel the quality of your Chi there. Feel your perineum opening, smiling and breathing in positive energy from the outside. Imagine that this place has a very sophisticated *filter* that can only allow in the best energy. Breathe as much as you can there, opening and smiling at your perineum. Be aware of the attributes of elemental Earth—unconditional support, nurturing, comfort, stability, consistency, balance, good perspective, fairness, regularity, rhythm, harmony—and associate them with that sense of support through your breathing and smiling perineum.

- Keep feeling the power of Earth at your perineum and smile in your tailbone, your sacrum, your genitals, and sexual center, together. Make them smile and open, feel them supported by the Earth power from the perineum. Bring a feeling of breathing with the sense of the powerful energy filter from there, and cultivate the feelings of balance and momentum in your sacrum, and creativity and life enjoyment in your sexual center. Sit and relax there for a while. Let these feelings build before you get to the next set of energy centers.

- Once you clearly feel these three centers open and supported by the elemental Earth attributes of comfort, unconditional support, and nurturing, along with the sense of momentum in your sacrum and creativity in your sexual center, bring your mind to your navel and Door of Life. Feel life force there and relax your back against it. Feel your navel and Door of Life equipped with their reliable filters. Feel them opening and smiling, breathing in positive energy from the outside without fear. Keep building the feelings of strength from your perineum, sacrum, sexual center, Door of Life, and navel for a while until they gather a momentum of their own.

Note to Practitioners: What are the filters referred to here? These are spiritual filters, meaning that our spirit is so well trained to have them shut, so we don't perceive anything that our energy level couldn't handle. When we finally perceive something through them, we can assume that the safety margin is huge. These filters are indeed very reliable.

- Next, feel the opening of your solar plexus and T11 opposite each other. Smile there, breathe through their filters, and cultivate the feelings of being able to change perspective and direction from your back, and the ability to appreciate and respect all perspectives from your solar plexus.

- Then, move to your heart center and T4 opposite each other and feel the opening, the smiling, and the breathing, with an inner sense of freedom and appreciation for life.

- Keep feeling the support of the Earth force from your perineum, momentum and creativity from your sacrum and sexual center, increased life force from your Door of Life and navel, freedom of movement and respect for different perspectives from your T11 and solar plexus, and liberation and appreciation for life from your heart and T4.

- Next, activate your throat center and C7 at the base of your neck between your shoulder blades and feel the ability to reach out and express yourself developing from there. Breathe and smile from there, and let the energy rise to your Jade Pillow, at the base of your skull, and connect directly to your mid-eyebrow. Open a big smile there. Breathe freely through the imaginary filters there and connect inwardly to that inner space, relaxing in free perception, in absolute effortless contemplation.

- Smile from the top of your head and open yourself to breathing and listening from there, trusting your filters and the unconditional support of the earth from your perineum.

- Feel all your centers open, smiling and breathing at the same time, getting in touch with the meaning and functions of each one. Stay there as long as you are comfortable.

CHAPTER ★ 6

Mapping the Emotional Body

Every part of the body has a function, which has a meaning for the emotional self. Although that meaning is partially defined by our belief system, I have found it to be fairly consistent across similar cultural backgrounds. Our bodies function similarly for good reasons. The whole of humanity usually suffers more or less from the same issues, and more or less seeks the same things in terms of enjoyment of life.

In my experience, the more an energetic charge manifests itself toward the front of the body, the more current the corresponding issue, and the more toward the back of the body, the more ancient the issues—sometimes even pre-birth related, such as family matters passed down through the bloodline. Pre-birth issues have been called past lives issues, cultural karma, and inner ghosts in many cultures, but for our purposes we can assume they are atavistic forces and heredity, or traumas resulting from dogmas, social and religious conditioning, and other matter carried by the collective unconscious.

If we look at the body bilaterally, usually the right side refers to Yang—active, mentally dominant, directive, and logically oriented (even for left-handed people), while the left side usually refers to Yin—corresponding to the affective side of the body, the side of abstraction, and emotional orientation. Most of the time, but not consistently, we find male figures on the right and female figures on the left. In many Asian populations, though, they are reversed. This could be because Asians, in general, are more matriarchal and women have a more dominant role in terms of managing the family, while men have a more active role in emotional support. Even in the West, there is a whole spectrum from Yin to Yang for both men and women, so there can be a wide range of overlap: Some men are more Yin than some women, and some women are more Yang than some men. There are many instances of more matriarchal families where the mother is the provider and decision maker, and the father is the family emotional support. In this case, the father would be manifested on the left side and the mother on the right. There are also instances of single parents in which these aspects are interchangeable.

Every good artist who has drawn the human body knows that the personality of an individual is reflected in every physical aspect. The body is very consistent with a person's psychological profile, and every part of the physical body will possess this undeniable quality. This is called *morphology*, the science of shapes. Thus, my toes are shaped the way they are because they are mine; to change the shape of my toes—and yes, it is possible—I have to change myself.

In light of this understanding, the following map is designed as a guide for you to make your own map for *every* client at *every* treatment.

Guide to the Body Map

It is of the utmost importance not to be dogmatic when mapping the emotional body. Every case is different and, as with maps, it's important to look at the terrain and make a map that fits the terrain instead of the other way around. So I will use the terms "usually" and "generally" very generously, and I would advise you to assume these terms even when I don't use them. Please test the terrain and don't be afraid to ask your client for accuracy and validation.

The Feet

Starting with the toes, I have noticed, with certain clients, how the shape of their toes changes after several Chi Nei Tsang sessions, even though I never work directly on their feet. Usually, after a few sessions the toes spread out, bunions regress, and the feet gain nearly a shoe size. To me, a bunion is an attempt by the body to grow an extra toe. When the big toe is free to move out from the other toes to stabilize the foot, bunions regress. But what is it in people that makes them hold their toes together and makes them prefer shoes that squeeze their toes? Toes and feet are for standing. Toes, like fingers, point to directions and are the extremities where energy extends. I believe that when people are constantly pointed in a certain direction in life, they develop pointed feet. When they are prevented from standing for themselves, and their spirit is strong, they develop foot problems as an internal conflict about the situation.

Case Study: Dancing Away the Pain

I have a client who developed a painful case of plantar fasciitis and was forbidden by her doctor to run or even walk too long. During her Chi Nei Tsang treatment, she understood that she had been "walking on eggshells." I suggested she stomp and take tap dance classes, which she had always wanted to do but couldn't because of the pain. The pain disappeared after that session, only to return during relationship problems with her dance instructor. She had thought that her pain resulted from dancing too hard, but apparently she hadn't been dancing hard enough. With a stronger emotional body, she went on to take more classes, including Flamenco and Latin dance. The pain never returned.

The Ankles

Ankles are designed to make the feet adapt to the nature of the ground they stand on, and, of course, the ground we stand on figuratively signifies the way we emotionally "stand up for" ourselves. I have found that ankles connect with adaptation and survival issues. Sometimes, during treatment, I ask clients to close their eyes and picture themselves standing. I let them describe what kind of ground they are standing on and how they feel. Is the ground solid or soft? Comfortable or rough? Is it rocky? Is it slippery or firm? Is it wet or dry? Is it slanted? Do both of their feet feel different? Answers to such questions make the emotional map more accurate.

The Knees

Knees take up the slack between the ankles and the hips, and are the articulations responsible for shock absorption and smoothness of walk. Figuratively speaking, without knees, we wouldn't have any protection from the roughness of life, and we would feel emotionally abandoned!

I have seen countless cases where knee problems were related to being orphaned literally, or symbolically, after the death of someone dear, after a breakup, or after psychological trauma—times and events when clients didn't feel validated by someone significant in their life, and they felt emotionally abandoned.

The Hips

Whether standing, kneeling, crawling, sitting, or even lying down, the hips are the basic support for the whole body. In the emotional body, they represent the parents. According to our belief system, we generally find issues related to our mothers on our left and paternal issues on our right.

The Sacrum and Coccyx

The sacrum, with the coccyx, is the center of momentum in life. When hit or injured, it can have a deep impact on our ability to fulfill our full life potential. Sacrum means "sacred" bone. This is the place where we hide our worst fears and terrors.

The Pelvis

Our pelvis is the place where life enjoyment resides. It is the location of sexual enjoyment but also of all kinds of enjoyment. It is important that the connection between our tailbone and sacrum, for momentum in life, and our pelvis be open and free so we can direct our life toward enjoyment and happiness.

The Lower Back and Kidneys

The lower back is where our kidneys are felt. This place is at L3, just opposite the navel. In Chinese, it is called Ming-Men, the "Door of Life." Our kidneys represent our inheritance in life potential. They contain our bank account of life currency. To relax here is to send the inner message that we don't have to worry, we can relax, we still have a lot to live on. To be tense here is to perpetually worry about the future.

T11

This is the vertebra that tilts and rotates, allowing us to change direction. Here we find issues connected with ability to change.

The Middle Back

The middle back, especially around T6, is responsible for holding our diaphragm with its ability to expand our breath and get us in touch with things we would rather not be aware of. T4 is right behind our heart and holds issues connected with freedom.

The Upper Back

The upper back, especially around C7, is responsible for connecting us with our arms and hands, and the ability to reach out, to exchange, to trade, to be in touch with ourselves, other people, and our surroundings at all levels—physical, mental, emotional, and spiritual. Being contracted here reflects being overwhelmed with responsibilities. Sometimes this place gets so tense that a hump develops here. This is commonly referred to as the Atlas syndrome, the feeling of holding the whole world on one's shoulders.

The Shoulders

This is the place where we hide emotionally. The right shoulder points to mental work and functional issues, and the left one points to emotional issues from which we are trying to hide.

The Neck

The neck is an extension of the upper back, and its main function is to direct the senses from the head without having to mobilize the whole body. Thus, the neck holds issues between responsibilities and awareness. Here we'll find all issues connected with control: self-control on the back of the neck, resisting control from others on the front of the neck, and issues of controlling others on the sides of the neck.

The Elbows

We use the elbows to protect ourselves from physical danger. When we are in danger, we instinctively raise our elbows. Pain in the elbows often connects with fear of receiving.

The Wrists

The wrists usually hold charges connected with giving.

The Fingers

They are the extension of our neck and upper back. They extend the Chi and are the places of connection between various meridians. Knowing about these meridians will help you understand the different issues connected with each finger.

The Forehead

Very often, the forehead holds charges connected with lying, culpability, and feeling responsible.

The Cheeks

They hold our smile and connect with having to hold appearances.

The Jaws

Emotionally charged jaws usually relate to victimization.

The Throat

This area is about being able to swallow emotional charges. The throat also connects with being able to express and verbalize these emotions. Throat issues might point to emotional charges that are not accepted and, therefore, cannot be validated.

The Ribs

Every rib, like every vertebra, has a personality and different charges attached to it. The most common ones are the front of rib 2, which holds charges connected with meeting expectations, and rib 6, where the diaphragm reaches the heart, connected with empathy and sharing feelings. Tensing rib 6 protects us from feeling too much.

The Sternum

The breastbone protects the heart and acts as a shield in front for the spirit. Holding our sternum high while *not* expanding the diaphragm at T6 expresses denial.

The Solar Plexus

The so-called pit of the stomach is actually a plexus of nerve fibers; it is the center of the felt sense, from pure physical sensation, to feelings, to emotions. When weak and held back, it manifests deep-seated emotional suffering. When protruding from the tightening of the upper part of the abdominal muscles, it expresses a need for emotional protection with a strong denial system.

The Digestive Tract

This tells us at what stage of digestion emotional charges are present. Emotions are the food of our soul. We have to swallow them, stomach them, take what we need out of them, and then eliminate what we don't need.

The Stomach and Duodenum

Here, we usually hold charges related to how we feel, and how we were made to feel about ourselves. Feelings of self-worth, self-consciousness, guilt, and shame will also be found here.

The Pancreas

The pancreas is the Yin Earth organ, where the most essential and most vital Earth issues reside. We see a frequent problem in this area among people who have been relocated, people who have lost their land and sense of identity, and among people who have been completely disconnected from all Earth principles and are not able to live in the present because the present is too uncomfortable. When Earth issues that are already present in the stomach and duodenum reach a chronic state, then hypoglycemia, and later diabetes, set in. Only systematic work on Earth issues can reverse this process.

The Liver

The liver is in charge of storing all non-water-soluble toxins and inorganic matter, whatever is difficult to metabolize, and extreme toxins such as heavy metals and toxic chemicals, in order to protect the rest of the body. Only when the liver has extra time and energy—which is rare—does it go through a detoxifying process, breaking down the chemicals into less toxic compounds to be evacuated via the kidneys, the skin, the lymphatic system, and the lungs. Figuratively speaking, the liver does the same thing with toxic emotions—emotions that we don't want to be in touch with, or emotions from which we want to protect others and ourselves. Once emotional charges are stored long enough, they tend to turn into anger for added protection. The liver secretes bile as its product; it is no coincidence that the word *bile* also signifies an inclination to anger.

The Gallbladder

The gallbladder takes the overflow of bile from the liver and concentrates it: it does the same with negative emotions. Once the liver is full, the gallbladder is in charge of taking that surplus and trying to store it. When negative emotions stagnate long enough in the liver, they turn into anger. We hold onto the anger with patience, to avoid "rocking the boat." This is when we form gallstones. There is no other reason to form and keep gallstones. Without the psychological profile of being patient and pretending not to be negatively affected, we would pass gallstones as soon as they formed, which is what happens all the time when we are healthy. Typically, gallstone clients have been through a long period with little laughter and a lot of stress. When they release their gallstones, painlessly and effortlessly during Chi Nei Tsang sessions, it is generally after connecting with some deep resentments.

The Diaphragm

This is the muscle of breath and feelings. We all breathe differently because we have different feelings. Awareness of feelings and emotions comes with awareness of breath. The diaphragm is a complex muscle. It is assisted by the intercostal muscles, between the ribs, to work out a strategy for breathing. A major part of a Chi Nei Tsang treatment is to allow clients to discover places within themselves where they have a hard time breathing, and thus discover places where emotional charges hide. Not surprisingly, in light of what we just said about the liver and its function of storing emotional charges, two-thirds of the liver is covered by the diaphragm. Our diaphragm is in direct relation to *all* our emotions, conscious or nonconscious.

The Lower Abdomen, Uterus, and Sacral Cavity

These are the places where the Wood energy grows generative and creative power, and where fecundation and pregnancy occur. It is also the place where excess Wood energy gets stored after the liver and gallbladder are filled up, and where it often manifests in women as fibroid tumors and endometriosis, and in men as prostate problems. This usually shows creative energy that is prevented from being used or is getting wasted in something unrelated or out of sync with our real-life purpose.

The Large Intestine

The large intestine is the last stage of emotional processing. It is the organ of emotional awareness. The large intestine, or colon, is quite long. The transverse segment hangs from both sides of the diaphragm at the phrenico-colic ligaments and has a major influence on breath, just as breath has a large influence on its functioning. At the cecum, the beginning of the large intestine, and the ascending colon, we hide issues we don't want to deal with. We don't want to know about them. Everything is obscure and undifferentiated. Then, as we progress toward the liver and the hepatic flexure, our awareness increases. After the transverse colon, the processing brings us to how we personally feel about it at the spleenic flexure, and by the time we pass the descending colon and reach the sigmoid colon, we know precisely what we are dealing with. But now the issue might be that we don't want others to know about it. So we find privacy-related issues and secrecy on the lower left side by the sigmoid colon.

PART ★ II

Emotional Healing Strategies, Techniques, and Prescriptions

CHAPTER ★ 7

Applications of the Universal Laws of Life to Our Mind and Emotions

Once we learn to juggle the laws of the Five Elemental Forces and have a better understanding of the principles of health—how we feel and think according to our energy pattern in general—our pattern of tensions and the health of our internal organs start to make sense. Clients become more predictable because practitioners know that they feel and think according to the health of their internal organs. It is important to understand this before we can heal and change. First we need to know what needs to be changed and feel it. As Moshe Feldenkrais used to say in his classes on awareness of movement, "You can't get what you want if you don't know what you do."

We, in Western culture, have learned through our educational system that rational thinking should dominate our mind, body, and spirit. The basic tenets of psychology stipulate that we think before we have emotions. We perceive, at the most, only two mental aspects: rational thinking and emotions. Both are qualified as mental—"in your head"—and have placed a dualistic perspective on human behavior: Either it is clear and logical, and originates at the mental level, or it comes from the shadows of the different layers of the unconscious mind. The inability to recognize our emotions, our denial, is mostly attributed to a lack of mental capacity.

According to Taoist perspective, we have neither one nor two but five mental aspects. These mental aspects stem from the Five Elemental Forces, and only when these five aspects work harmoniously do we have full mental capacity.

Plates 15 through 22 illustrate the general points made in this part of the chapter.

Mental Aspects and the Law of Creation

Plate 23 relates the law of creation with mental aspects and both positive and negative emotions.

Wood: I Think, Therefore I Am

As we learned in Chapter 2, Water nurtures Wood. Once we attain a good amount of power with Water, our Wood grows in a healthy manner. This means that our ability to be creative with Water will feed our rational thinking. Abstraction and dreams feed our ability to discover and understand. The same way that the tree, the symbol of Wood, is a complete ecosystem, our rational mind, our intelligence, creates our own universe.

Fire: I Know, Therefore I Am

Once we understand (Wood), our wisdom (Fire) leads us to believe and to know. We then have a strong sense of guidance toward our life purpose; we call it intuition. Intuition is our highest level of intelligence. It is the complete growth process of Wood culminating in the bloom (Fire). This also means that our intuition is proportional to our level of mental cultivation. If our intelligence is low, we can't expect our intuition to be any higher. There is no shortcut in education. Only discipline, training, and consistent work can enable our Wood energy and intelligence to bloom into intuition, wisdom, and the spiritual guidance that tells us what to do, what our heart wants, and what makes us happy and gives us enthusiasm for life.

Earth: I Do, Therefore I Am

Once we know (Fire), then we feel happy and comfortable, and we can enjoy the fruits of having a secure foundation and a good perspective on life (Earth). This allows us to manifest the right idea at the right time, at the right place, for the right purpose, with the right people. This is what is meant by being clever, spontaneous, and practical. We can then enjoy a strong sense of authenticity with a solid appreciation for life on Earth and behave effortlessly and comfortably with a sense of purpose.

Metal: I Feel, Therefore I Am

Only when we stand on the firm ground of recognition and validation (Earth), and are solid enough to get that clear perspective on life, can we afford to be sensitive enough (Metal) to have the courage to face the nonrationality and immediacy of our feelings, to grow from them and be emotionally mature. Only then can we be completely honest with ourselves and with others, and be on good terms with our emotional life, the very fabric of our soul.

Water: I Dream, Therefore I Am

Once we feel our emotions (Metal), then we dream (Water) about them. Our dreams feed on the abstraction of our emotional life, from the bottom of which creativity, vision, and willpower emerge. In Water is also our instinct that makes us react without thinking. Water carries the original information, the idea that will be developed and cultivated in Wood. Creativity waters the growth of our mental cultivation (Wood) and turns it into clarity.

With further cultivation, more fragrant and colorful blooms produce more delicious fruits as the upward spiral of refinement continues. This is the principle of internal alchemy held sacred by Taoists monks and Chi-Kung practitioners.

Starting with Yin Water, the most Yin, the deepest, most hidden and essential manifestation of our thinking process, is our ability to be creative, to conceive of and summon new ideas from the depths of our psyche from the abstraction of our dream world. Creativity is our mental Water aspect. Next, our mind grows fully formed thoughts in the Wood mental aspect of intelligence, with our ability to develop theories, make plans, and create strategies for solving problems. Our mind then blooms into the Fire mental aspects of wisdom, spirit, and guidance. We are then able to use the right idea, at the right place, at the right time with Earth, thus making practicality and spontaneity the Earth mental aspects. Great awareness of emotions comes out of this Earth support, thereby becoming the mental aspect in Metal, allowing us to outgrow these emotions and to become a better and more mature self.

If our energy is high, all goes well and the cycle of creation nourishes our mind in a productive way. But when our basic life force weakens, there is a lack of Chi in our Water system (kidneys and adrenals); we become tired, we are not very creative, and our thinking becomes fuzzy (Wood). Our spirit is then disheartened (Fire), we have a tendency to lose perspective on things (Earth), and we become quite insensitive and depressed (Metal).

Emotional Aspects and the Law of Creation

When our energy is low or stagnant, we experience the negative aspects of our mind. Likewise, when we are refreshed and relaxed, and our energy runs abundantly, we experience the positive aspects of our mind. These are all natural reactions. It is pure physics. Remember, we don't choose our feelings; we get them. If we had the choice, we would go for what feels good! Forcing ourselves to "think positively," "smile," or "just forgive and forget" means forcing our thinking process to overcome our emotions, which is impossible. Metal cuts Wood (see the next section on the law of control). Only in cases where the mind is so strong and the emotional charge very weak or mostly outgrown, can Wood overpower Metal. What happens is that, in most cases, we force ourselves to become numb and hide the emotional charges in parts of our body that we have to alienate from ourselves to avoid feeling bad. This is the legitimate thing to do since we were originally born to *enjoy* life, not to *suffer*. But we can never really forget these emotions hidden within ourselves; all our nervous system can do for us is to try to not remember!

In scientific approaches, as well as in Taoism, there is no moral judgment involved when we talk of "positive" and "negative" emotions. Positive and negative are understood at the strictly energetic level: in physics there is nothing wrong with the negative pole of a battery and nothing especially good about the positive pole. It is all a matter of magnetic charge. Similarly, with emotions, when the energy is low or stagnant, we experience negative emotions, and when the energy runs healthily and abundantly, we experience positive feelings.

Let's start with Water, extreme Yin, even though there is no real beginning or end to the cycle.

Water

The emotional force of Metal nourishes the emotional force of Water.

Positive emotions: If Water energy is plentiful, we feel full of life force, and we have so much energy to spend, that we have to be calm and gentle. There is no need to rush or to rev up the engine. We can just follow the momentum since it is so strong. It is much like a large but calm river that flows swiftly, compared to a little stream that appears to be rushing. Our great awareness and the courage to face our emotions, and the uprightness and pride in Metal, allow for great calm, originality, and a great outflow of effortless power in the creative energy of Water.

Negative emotions: Let's assume that energy is running so low that the basic life force is dropping. Since Water is the most Yin, most essential element for life, the feeling connected with losing it is fear. This is legitimate, and there is nothing wrong about feeling afraid when we feel weaker than a given situation would require. If we feel too weak to run from the beast, then extreme terror arises. If we know that we can outrun the situation, just a small amount of fear is all that is necessary to make us run a little faster.

The phenomenon of paralysis and numbness from terror is a necessary reaction in nature so that animals can naturally succumb to predators without suffering. The energy that would be used to run away turns inwardly to paralyze and numb the victim. In the context of weakness and negative emotional charges, depression, sadness, and grief in Metal will provoke weak will in Water, leading to fear and paranoid tendencies.

Wood

The emotional force of Water nourishes the emotional force of Wood.

Positive emotions: If the energy from Water is strong and feeds us with plenty of calm, then we are going to grow a lot of kindness and generosity in Wood. When a tree is abundant with ripe fruit, it has to let the fruit drop. There is no other choice—if it doesn't, the fruit rots on the tree, and the whole tree then rots and dies. When we are wealthy (money, knowledge, wisdom, skills), we need to circulate that wealth and share it so that we, too, don't rot and die with it!

Negative emotions: If we are afraid in Water, and that fear is feeding our Wood, frustration and anger are going to grow in Wood. There is nothing wrong with this. If we are subjected to abuse, dispossession, and submission, we will react with anger. This is a healthy reaction. Anger is a surface emotion (Yang) that raises power and protects us from feeling the underlying emotions of sadness, grief, and fear, which would paralyze us and rob us of the energy necessary to respond to the situation if we let ourselves feel them.

Fire

The emotional force of Wood nourishes the emotional force of Fire.

Positive emotions: If we have strength and calm in Water, it will grow into so much wealth that we have to be generous and kind in Wood so that we can be joyous and happy in Fire. We are successful, and we can enjoy it.

Negative emotions: If we grow anger in Wood, then we'll eventually explode into absolute impatience and hatred in Fire. We just can't take it anymore; it is time for change. We can then become completely insensitive (because Fire melts Metal—again, see the next section on the law of control), slashing, burning, and killing without a second thought. This would be a natural reaction.

Earth

The emotional force of Fire nourishes the emotional force of Earth.

Positive emotions: If we are calm in Water, kind and generous in Wood, and are happy and enjoy a high spirit in Fire, we can then enjoy emotional stability, fairness, and good perspective in Earth. This allows us to be practical, present, authentic, and spontaneous.

Negative emotions: If we live with impatience and hatred in our heart (Fire), we won't feel good or comfortable experiencing the present moment. Instead, we will feel like hurrying. We'll feel like the world is inhospitable, and that we are standing on shaky ground. It is hard to feel good about ourselves under such conditions, when we feel rejected by earth and existence. From here, poor self-esteem, worries, and chronic anxiety arise.

Metal

The emotional force of Earth nourishes the emotional force of Metal.

Positive emotions: If the energy coming from Earth is strong, solid, and abundant, and we feel comfortable, accepted, validated, and allowed to really be ourselves and are proud of it; likewise, if we experience high spirit and joy from Fire, clarity of mind and kindness in Wood, and strength and calm in Water, we can afford to have the courage to face the deepest, darkest, most unpleasant sides of ourselves in Metal. This is true honesty and takes courage, uprightness, and pride. It takes these kinds of emotions to let ourselves feel intensely and completely. This is why healing at the emotional level is so difficult. We won't heal if we are prevented from developing our emotional and mental aspects. We won't have the strength to face our hidden selves.

Negative emotions: If we stand on shaky ground in Earth, we will feel like looking for protection and advantages even though our very condition prevents us from having a good perspective on things. We are "out of touch" (Metal), so we'll experience confusion in our feelings. We will be unfair and biased and are in no condition to be honest with ourselves or with others. We'll make mistakes by looking for protection through what is most convincing rather than by what is real, trusting appearances rather than reality. Sadness, melancholy, and nostalgia, at best, are all that we can feel, but numbness and depression are the result of our not being able to let ourselves feel emotional at all.

Mental Aspects If Energy Is Positive and Abundant

Plates 16 through 18 illustrate the points about mental and emotional aspects. "Healthy" and "weak" describe the energy of the overall organ system. For example, weak Kidney energy, which causes fear, means that if we have weak kidneys, we will have a propensity for being scared, and being scared all the time will eventually weaken the kidneys. By "Kidney," we not only mean the kidneys, but also the bones, the marrow, the teeth, the ears, the Kidney and Bladder meridian system, and the DNA.

Water (healthy Kidney energy): inspired, creative, inventive, insightful, original, dynamic, productive.

Wood (healthy Liver energy): thoughtful, intelligent, clear, articulate, cultivated, prosperous, progressive, constructive, open-minded, curious, always ready to learn more.

Fire (healthy Heart and Endocrine energy): bright, high-spirited, humorous, spiritual, respectful, humble, reverent, virtuous, intuitive.

Earth (healthy Spleen-Pancreas energy): aware, practical, smart, content, satisfied, balanced, good judgment, good taste, present, authentic, conciliatory.

Metal (healthy Lung energy): emotionally intelligent, very sharp, nonjudgmental, sensual, playful, sociable, refined.

Mental Aspects If Energy Is Negative and/or Deficient

Plate 19 illustrates the negative mental aspects.

Water (weak Kidney energy): slow, tired, weak, uninventive.

Wood (weak Liver energy): limited, stubborn, dogmatic, obsessive.

Fire (weak Heart and Endocrine energy): stern, dark, secretive, severe.

Earth (weak Spleen-Pancreas energy): dissatisfied, gluttonous or restrained, austere, disproportionate, disharmonized, tasteless, artificial, unfair, prejudiced, desynchronized, unfriendly, inhospitable.

Metal (weak Lung energy): dull, out of touch, timid, dishonest, biased, artificial.

Emotional Aspects If Energy Is Positive and Abundant

Continuing to refer to Plate 19, positive and abundant energy has the following emotional aspects.

Water (healthy Kidney energy): calm, gentle, embracing, limitless, encompassing, determined, creative, sensual.

Wood (healthy Liver energy): generous, patient, kind, tempered, cool-headed, pleasant, discreet, relaxed, cooperative.

Fire (healthy Heart and Endocrine energy): joyful, warm, compassionate, spiritual, hearty, respectful, polite, patient, loving, forgiving, unconditional, passionate, enthusiastic.

Earth (healthy Spleen-Pancreas energy): fair, empathic, supportive, solid, consistent, congenial, spontaneous, genuine, harmonious, centered, rooted, stable, balanced, solid, healthy in appetite and desires, regular, harmonized, synchronized, sociable, hospitable, nurturing, comfortable, ease of being, easygoing.

Metal (healthy Lung energy): courageous, cool, firm, uplifted, resonant, pure, pardoning, forgiving, upfront, true to one's feelings, upright, proud, honest.

Emotional Aspects If Energy Is Negative and/or Deficient

Plate 19 illustrates the emotional aspects found in the face of negative or deficient energy.

Water (weak Kidney energy): afraid, rough, cold, slippery, small, scattered, speedy, stagnant, running in circles, boring, sterile, tedious, lewd, paranoid.

Wood (weak Liver energy): angry, frustrated, aggressive, stingy, violent, sly, hot-headed, explosive, obstreperous, tight, obsessed, obstinate, formalistic, utopian, competitive, antagonistic, arrogant, thoughtless, petty, jealous, resentful.

Fire (weak Heart and Endocrine energy): impatient, hateful, spiteful, vicious, cruel, cynical, inconsiderate, mocking, insensitive, obsequious.

Earth (weak Spleen-Pancreas energy): anxious, awkward, imbalanced, inconsistent, absent, intrusive, worried, shaky, envious, jealous, low self-esteem, unreliable, irresponsible.

Metal (weak Lung energy): reactive, hypocritical, cowardly, hesitant, treacherous, deceitful, sad, depressed, emotionally confused, unsure.

Emotional and Mental Aspects and the Law of Control

Using the law of control, we can change undesirable emotional patterns, controlling negative feelings (see Plate 24).

Now, what do we do if we feel a certain way that we don't like feeling, and we want to change? It is clear that no amount of understanding will change much of the condition. We are aware that these unpleasant feelings result from energetic charges that are difficult or impossible to digest. We know that these emotional charges affect our physical self, according to the function of that physical aspect of ourselves. What we need next is a system of guidance to help process these charges efficiently. This will first involve our mental functions to validate the feelings in order to give permission for the growth process and change to take place. Second, physical touch might be necessary to help stimulate our system and guide the negative charges into complete processing and elimination.

WATER

Controlling Excess Fear: Building and Strengthening Our Earth
Transforming Fear into Calm and Creativity

If our energy runs low or is congested in our Kidney-Bladder energetic system, we experience feelings of fear. If we look at Plate 25, showing the elemental universal laws of nature, we see that Earth controls Water. The mental aspects of Earth are awareness, practicality, and spontaneity. Practical awareness is a bridge to clarity and logic and will help counteract the irrationality of excess fear by bringing a sense of perspective, and some feeling of solidity, stability, and safety in the here and now.

- Fear extinguishes joy and enthusiasm from our Heart (Fire).
- Metal sensitivity can only turn our fear (Water) into a flood.
- No amount of explanation (Wood) can sufficiently calm our fear.
- Only by being aware, by seeing that at least, here and now, in the present (Earth), everything is okay, can we calm down.

Strong Earth holds Water. Mental stability counteracts excess fear. Strengthening our Earth attributes consists of:

- Attending to our home and sense of comfort.
- Following the Three Laws of Dietary Hygiene (see *Healing from Within,* p. 148) on a regular basis.
- Practicing the Earth Chi-Kung exercises and meditations.

This will eventually provide us with enough stability, solidity, and balance so that chronic fears can evaporate from our Water system.

Wood

Controlling Excess Anger: Sharpening and Polishing Our Metal
Transforming Anger into Kindness and Generosity

Anger is a very important emotion, but it is also frightening, so we have a tendency to hide it from ourselves and from others. A Wood attribute, anger comes with thinking and planning. It arises spontaneously when things don't go as planned. Since it also comes from our liver, the main internal organ of the Wood system, it also means that when our liver is congested or overwhelmed with toxicity or pollutants, we can't help but feel hostile. A certain level of hostility is so frequent among some of us that it is now considered "normal." We have no idea how much hostility we carry, and how detrimental our chronic anger is to our own health. This anger always underlies our activities, especially our leisure, games, and pastimes. It is easily apparent in our sports, our favorite shows that contain some sort of violence, the use of weapons and explosives, and by our propensity for seeking scapegoats or competitors to blame for difficulties.

When this happens, there is no amount of reasoning possible because to do so requires clarity of mind (Wood), which is completely immobilized by its negative emotional aspect, aggressiveness. This actually makes us very sharp "intellectuals," who constantly find reasons to justify the way we feel. Remember, Metal cuts Wood. The only way out of the escalation of violence is to stop thinking and start breathing! Only deep breathing can bring us back in touch with the nonrational, but nevertheless very important emotional level and appreciation for life, which is lost with excessive thinking. Once positive feelings are pumped back into the lungs (Metal), anger (Wood) transforms itself into its positive counterparts, kindness and generosity (see Plate 26).

Fire

Controlling Impatience and Insensitivity: Channeling Water, Controlling Fire
Transforming Impatience into Enthusiasm

Driving fast or walking fast without being in a hurry, even under the pretense of having fun, is one of the main symptoms of undetected emotional Fire imbalance and inner impatience. Often, impatience and insensitivity are a result of excess Wood over-fueling Fire, a side effect of denied anger feeding insensitivity and impatience. Cutting Wood with Metal can help, but sometimes the Fire is burning so intensely that no amount of breathing can extinguish the fire of derision and cruelty. In fact, breathing will make it even stronger; it will make us laugh! The Fire has to be controlled by Water (see Plate 27). Fear, of course, can put a damper on our over-impatient and hasty Fire element by frightening us with the prospect of punishment. However, from a more positive aspect, stimulating and cultivating creativity and sensuality, providing a safe and hospitable place (Earth) where creativity (Water) can be channeled, will progressively transform impatience and hastiness into high spirit and enthusiasm.

EARTH

Controlling Chronic Anxiety and Poor Self-Esteem: Cultivating Our Wood Intelligence
Transforming Anxiety into Solidity and Ease of Being

Anxiety is a sign of weak Earth, like standing on shaky ground (see Plate 28). When Earth is low, it is easily flooded with Water, which is why anxiety and fear are very closely related. In addition to fear, poor self-esteem comes with weak Earth, which is what differentiates it from a Water imbalance.

I have noticed that anywhere the land has been exploited, over-industrialized, mined, or drilled for oil, the quality of Earth Chi feels depleted. I have also noticed that people living there are usually not very hospitable and look very submissive and angry. Even people working in shops, hotels, and restaurants in these areas don't feel like investing in qualities that will attract and maintain a clientele, and they lose business as a result. I believe that we become anxious and scared when we don't feel supported by Earth. Unconsciously, we become hostile and, of course, look for and find all kinds of reasons to be that way. There is a noticeable difference, for example, in regions where a national park or a nature preserve has been established on landfill or a former dump site. As soon as you step through the gate of the park, a positive energy charge is instantly felt.

On the other hand, the reverse is felt in certain zones of power all over the earth. For example, where I live, there is a hill that feels extremely calm. Even the shopping mall on top of the hill is calm and quiet. I find the shopkeepers and clerks there more easygoing and pleasant than in any other shopping mall I have ever patronized. One day, I even took a nap in the parking lot! It is so calm that the management decided to relocate the movie theaters and the car dealers to the next hill because they felt they could do better business there. I believe that the original hill must contain some strongly positive telluric force or perhaps it was a sacred place for earlier civilizations and still carries that residual energetic charge.

If you would like to raise the quality of the Earth energy near you or where you live, all you have to do is practice Earth Chi-Kung and meditations on a regular basis. Another good technique is to visit your favorite powerful places on earth—your personal places of power, your favorite lookout over the ocean, your favorite mountain, the Grand Canyon, Monument Valley, Mount Shasta, shrines, monasteries, temples and churches—and bring the positive feelings from these places back to where you live, and to places where the earth feels depleted, and meditate and exercise there. This really works!

A very effective way to transform an Earth imbalance in yourself is by cultivating your Wood intelligence. Study, learn a new language or craft, learn to play an instrument, or do anything to stimulate your nervous system, to open your mind, and raise your spirit.

Metal

Controlling Depression: Elevating Our Spirit and Kindling Inner Fire
Transforming Sadness into Courage, Honesty, and Pride

I have heard it said so often and in so many ways: "I was saved ..." by Jesus, by Mary, by the Goddess, by Allah, by Buddha, by the Tao, by my guru, by God. These are examples of religion saving people from deep depression, the angst of existential anxiety, and from suicidal tendencies. Religion, however, must first feed the spirit and raise it to a level of being where we are in touch with our life purpose. This doesn't mean, though, that the only way out of depression is to join the first religious group or local cult available. Indeed, for some of us, this would have exactly the opposite effect.

What is important is to raise the spirit, and this can be accomplished through various means. Norman Cousins, well known for documenting his own healing by filming himself being treated for terminal cancer, discovered the way to salvation and complete remission through laughter.[10] He would get videos of his favorite comedians and watch them all day long, forcing himself to laugh. Some of us have achieved the same result by playing laugh-along audio recordings. We have even formed laughing clubs and associations, meeting every morning before work to exchange a few jokes and coax each other to laugh for several minutes every day. My main Chi-Kung master, Mantak Chia, has made Laughing Chi-Kung a regular part of his practice.

Yet, for others, raising our spirit requires completely different means. Again, we are all different, and these differences have to be respected in order to come up with something genuine and authentic so that we can overcome depression, and rekindle our enthusiasm for life.

One form of depression, which is very common in affluent countries, stems from having too many options, too many possibilities, too much choice, too many liberties, not *to have to do* anything with our life. We have tried different religions, different self-help programs, have traveled everywhere, and seen all the movies and comedies. Yet, we still have no taste for life because our spirit is low. We don't know what to do with ourselves. We have lost, or never acquired, our sense of purpose or destiny. Some of us are faced with the opposite, being prevented from realizing ourselves due to economic or prejudicial reasons.

Again, this is not about looking for solutions. We are faced here with something that *has no solution*. The only way out of emotional distress is not to try to solve anything, but to outgrow the situation. Literally, growing out of it means digesting it, being able to take in what we need and eliminate what we don't. Each of these reactions is, in fact, a healthy reaction to an unhealthy situation. Anyone placed in the same situation would experience the same thing or even worse. The way out of emotional distress is emotional maturity, which requires having undergone emotional episodes and survived. (See Plate 29.)

Note to Practitioners: The job of the practitioner working with a depressed client is not to find a solution or remedy, but to train the client into feeling *more* instead of less, by widening the spectrum of feelings. Only systematic exercises in deep breathing and meditation can do this. These will usually bring the person to the bottom of depression (the price of awareness), but also eventually to breakthrough (the reward). This is very hard to do and requires strength, determination, and experience as well as unconditional mental and emotional support from the practitioner.

Easy Breathing Chi-Kung[11]

If you feel like you don't have any control over your breath, if the very idea of a breathing exercise seems overwhelming, then this exercise is for you. I actually recommend that everyone start any breathing exercise with this one, even, and especially, if you are in the middle of an asthma attack! This exercise will help you calm down your breath and rapidly oxygenate your system with a minimal amount of effort.

The principle of this exercise is not to focus on the in-breath at all, but to emphasize the out-breath by progressively getting rid of residual, stagnant air from your lungs. This exercise consists of exhaling in three or four stages without any in-breath in between.

Practice very gently without getting out of breath, even if your breath is very shallow. Your lung capacity will improve rapidly with gentle practice every day.

- In any position—sitting, standing, or lying down—relax your shoulders and your chest by shaking them gently and letting them drop as much as possible without forcing. Be aware of the weight of your sternum and your ribs and let them drop.

- Let your body rock or sway slowly throughout the practice to avoid stiffness and to help release stagnant energies.

- Keep swaying calmly while breathing out.

- Pause without inhaling. Relax. Block your nose and mouth so you don't breathe in.

- Breathe out some more without forcing.

- Pause again, relax more, swallow your saliva to relax your chest and throat further, but make sure you don't inhale.

- Breathe out more even if it is just a little.

- Let yourself inhale and be aware of how much more than usual you can breathe without forcing.

- If you are out of breath after this exercise, let yourself recuperate and breathe normally for a few breaths and practice more easily and gently until you no longer get out of breath.

- Try to relax as much as possible by letting your body weight sink deeper into gravity and breathe out again one nice long out-breath without forcing.

- Then pause, don't inhale, and breathe out some more.

- Pause, and again breathe out some more, and pause one more time, and then squeeze out all the residual air left from your lungs.

- And let yourself breathe in again.

- Keep breathing in and out for a while until your breath is calm. Then repeat the cycle a dozen times.

This exercise will work best if done without hurrying or forcing. When you first start practicing the Easy Breathing Chi-Kung, it is okay—even better, perhaps—that you feel you are doing it poorly. Don't practice hard, but practice often. As with most Chi-Kung practices, the benefits come more from frequency rather than from intensity of effort.

If you have asthma or emphysema, practice regularly two or three times at first, and build up to six times daily. It will help you cope more easily when in crisis and reduce your number of episodes.

Prescribing Arts and Crafts for Emotional Healing

The arts and professions are associated with mental, emotional, and spiritual health. Arts can balance our professional choices. Plate 30 shows these associations.

We are usually drawn to the profession that matches our psychological profile, because it increases or justifes, and thus anchors, our natural tendencies and imbalances. In most cases, however, it is not necessary to change professions. We are better at what we do than anyone else because we enjoy what we do. Changing professions would only bring grief and add to the stress response. What is important is not to change the profession, but rather to change the accompanying mental and emotional attitudes. These attitudes can radically transform when aided by practicing at leisure the art corresponding to the controlling element. Of course, it is important that such art be practiced with its corresponding mental and emotional attributes. However, it is common that after going through healing, we find it necessary to change careers. Then, of course, we would naturally be attracted to activities that support our personal evolution and healing process.

Water

Professions: commerce, finance, diplomatic corps, travel, consulting.

Arts: figurative arts—painting, drawing, and sculpture, as well as photography and film—bring the essence of life to figures and manifest the power of abstraction and dreams.

If you are dominated by Water, you will usually be attracted to and be successful in the fields of finance and commerce. When plagued by a Water imbalance (excessive fearfulness, paranoia, irrational terrors), you might want to cultivate a taste for gardening, horticulture, or building or fixing something in order to exercise your ability to be practical and ingenious, and to develop a taste for stability, solidity, nurturing, and harmony.

Wood

Professions: military, law enforcement, firefighting, paramedics, politics, legal professions, management, clerical work, academics, science, psychology, physics, environmental studies, and all specialized professions.

Arts: writing in general, poetry, and martial arts.

If you are dominated by Wood, you might do very well working in the field of management, the sciences, the legal profession, politics, the military, and any field involving strategy. If you have a Wood imbalance (daydreaming, insomnia, obsessions, chronic anger, alcoholism), find solace in learning to play an instrument, listening intensely to music, or involving yourself in the esthetics of fashion, clothing, jewelry, and cosmetics to get in touch with your emotional life without the need for understanding or justifying.

Fire

Professions: teachers, doctors, spiritual leaders, priests, monks, gurus, physicians, herbalists.

Arts: performing arts—dance, singing, mime, acting, theatre, opera, drama, comedy.

Fire-dominated people often work as doctors, healers, teachers, trainers, and spiritual leaders. With a Fire imbalance (always in a rush, impatient, insensitive), you can find peace in painting, photography, sculpting, and the like, and cultivating your dream life by maintaining a dream journal (Water).

Earth

Professions: architecture, construction, carpentry, masonry, electrical contracting, plumbing, engineering, antiques dealing, agriculture, horticulture, gardening and landscaping, restoration, farming, fishing, hunting.

Arts: all artisans crafts—knitting, shoemaking, tailoring, jewelry making, furniture building, pottery, weaving, and cooking and all culinary and domestic arts.

Earth-dominated people can often be found as artisans, construction workers, farmers, hoteliers, or restaurateurs. If you have an Earth imbalance (uncomfortable, dissatisfied, poor self-esteem), you can find support, and start to learn about satisfaction, through Wood-related activities such as writing, reading, or martial arts. Additionally, you would benefit from any type of study that improves mental capacities such as foreign languages, mathematics, physics, astrology, botany, anthropology, history, and geography.

Metal

Professions: perfumers, trend-oriented professions, publicists, fashion and other designers, couturiers, estheticians.

Arts: music, the art of summoning feelings from pure abstraction.

If dominated by Metal, you are in touch with trends, esthetics, appearance, and health, and will do well working in any of these fields. Your Metal imbalance (depression, grief, sadness, and melancholy) can be relieved through dance, singing, chanting, and getting in touch with spirituality (Fire). Also you will find relief by strengthening old friendships or building new ones, adopting a pet, and finding love.

~~~~~~

Fusion of the Five Elements (Short Version): Recycling Negative Feelings into Positive Energy

This version of the Fusion of the Five Elements meditation is a very abridged version designed for Chi Nei Tsang practitioners to practice while giving treatments. It helps to trigger the full Fusion practice as taught by Taoist Master Mantak Chia and his lineage of teachers. This short version will start the process for practitioners who haven't yet had the chance to attend the full Fusion of the Five Elements class. Master Chia's Fusion of the Five Elements is the subject of an entire book,[13] and is taught as a weeklong retreat. The Fusion of the Five Elements meditation is the most healing practice I know. The power acquired from this meditation is applied directly to Chi Nei Tsang treatments.

- Sit in a comfortable position with your back erect but not stiff.

- Take the time for a thorough inner smile bath (*Healing from Within*, p. 273) while breathing gently.

- Breathe calmly, centering your breath behind your navel, making sure that you are still breathing into your sacrum and pelvic floor, lower back, lateral sides of your rib cage, and all the way inside your shoulder blades. Go back to the Easy Breathing Chi-Kung if you feel any breathing resistance.

- Behind your navel, build an empty sphere and let that sphere expand as you inhale and contract as you exhale. Make sure that your sphere stays right behind your navel. Don't let it go upward during inhalations. Make sure it remains a perfect sphere, and that it doesn't pull more to one side or the other.

- Take some time on your sphere. Make sure it is completely empty. It is neither dark nor clear; it is a completely empty sphere of pure vacuum.

- Be aware of the presence of heat inside your body. You are going to scan your whole body, gathering all the feelings of heat you can find into a red-hot sphere that you are going to hold in the middle of your chest right behind your sternum.

- Go around your whole body and take the time to locate the places where you feel heat. It might be in your head, certain places in your back, your neck, in your blood, anywhere inside your body.

- Pick up these feelings of heat from wherever you feel them, gather them into a red-hot ball—very red, very hot—and keep that ball or sphere securely in the middle of your chest.

- Go deep within yourself and gather all the feelings of impatience you can find. Pick up these feelings from wherever you feel them. Drag them and put them into that sphere behind your chest, where it feels very hot and very red, and keep them securely there.

- Now you feel the heat in your chest, very clear and very distinct, with all your impatience there.

- Next, be aware of the presence of cold inside your body. Scan your whole body, gathering all the feelings of cold you can find into a deep blue sphere that you are going to hold in your lower abdomen.

- Go around your whole body and take the time to locate the places where you feel cold. It might be in your back, in your sacrum, deep in your bones, anywhere inside your abdomen, or your chest, or your head.

- Pick up these feelings of cold and bring them into that sphere deep in your lower abdomen where it feels cold and dark. Make sure you put all your cold there and keep it there.

- Go deep within yourself and gather all the feelings of fear and terror you can find. Pick up these feelings from wherever they are and bring them into that deep, cold, dark sphere inside your lower abdomen. Put them there and keep them there.

- Now you feel all your cold in your lower abdomen, very clear and very distinct, with all your fear there.

- Also feel all your heat in the middle of your chest with all your impatience there and all your fear in your lower abdomen.

- Keep feeling all your heat and impatience in your chest and all your cold and fear in your lower abdomen, and be aware of that empty sphere behind your navel.

- Very slowly and carefully, take all the cold from your lower abdomen and bring it up the right side of your body to the middle of your chest and, at the same time, bring all your heat from the center of your chest down the left side of your body to your lower abdomen.

- Make sure that you bring these feelings all in one piece—all your heat and impatience down the left side of your body from your chest to your lower abdomen so there is no longer any heat felt in your chest, and all the cold and fear up the right side of your body from your lower abdomen to the middle of your chest so there is no more cold in your abdomen.

- Now feel the heat in your lower abdomen and the cold in the middle of your chest—very clear, very distinct—and be aware of the empty sphere behind your navel.

- Take all the cold from your chest and all the heat from your lower abdomen and pour them into that empty sphere and stir them together.

- Keep mixing and stirring all the cold and the heat, the red and the blue, using your mind's eye until that mixing and stirring gathers a momentum of its own.

- Now, under the right side of your rib cage, feel heat and dampness building into a dark green sphere.

- Feel heat and dampness gathering from all your nerves, all the tension and stress you may find there, dripping down into a dark green sphere that you are going to hold under the right side of your rib cage.

- Take the time to feel heat and dampness building under the right side of your rib cage—very hot and very damp, like a strong sauna, a steam bath, or a sweat lodge.

- Go deep within yourself and gather all the feelings of anger, hostility, frustration, and resentment you can find. Gather them into that dark, green sphere and keep them under the right side of your rib cage.

- Next, be aware of the left side of your rib cage. There, you are going to feel cold and dryness building into a bright white sphere.

- Feel a cold and dry wind blowing from the whole surface of your skin and from the depth of your lungs gathering into the bright white sphere under the left side of your rib cage.

- Go deep within yourself and gather all the feelings of sadness, grief, and depression you can find. Gather them into that bright white sphere under the left side of your rib cage and keep these feelings there.

- Now you feel cold and dryness under the left side of your rib cage with all your sadness there, and you feel the heat and dampness under the right side of your rib cage with all your anger there. Make it very clear and distinct.

- Keep feeling the heat and dampness on your right, and the cold and dryness on your left, and be aware of the sphere behind your navel where the heat and cold are still mixing together.

- Take all the heat and dampness from your right side, and all the cold and dryness from your left side, and pour them into the sphere behind your navel, mixing them together.

- Take your time and make sure there is no heat or dampness remaining under the right side of your rib cage and no cold and dryness under the left side of your rib cage. Feel them slowly mixing together in the sphere behind your navel. It might feel very thick and hard to mix at first, but keep working at it until it becomes easier and faster.

- Soon it doesn't feel so hot or so cold, it doesn't feel too damp or too dry. It starts to feel more comfortable and balanced. Keep the momentum of mixing and stirring going.

- Next, be aware of your solar plexus. Go deep within yourself and collect all feelings of uneasiness and discomfort you can find—all the feelings of self-consciousness, shame or guilt, the bad feelings you have about yourself or that you were made to feel about yourself, everything that feels unfair and unjust.

- Gather them from wherever they are and throw them directly inside the sphere behind your navel where everything is stirring and mixing together.

- Keep blending and stirring as if you were preparing a cake mix for baking, transforming it from something raw, rough, and unpleasant to something smooth, light, and fluffy.

- After a while, you will feel the mix getting very smooth and easy, starting to be perfectly blended. Not too hot, not too cold, not too damp, and not too dry, like perfectly balanced weather, or that cake mix, perfect for the oven.

- Let a feeling of balance and comfort expand inside your sphere behind your navel and make that sphere expand inside your body. Let it expand and let the feelings of ease and comfort spread inside your whole body.

- Feel it like perfect weather—lots of sunshine but not too hot, a little breeze but not too cold, a lot of grass but not damp. It feels very comfortable, very peaceful. Like an ideal place to rest, ideal weather and an ideal place for a picnic or a lazy stroll.

- Let that sphere spread and expand inside yourself—your whole abdomen, pelvis, and chest—and keep expanding until you find your whole self inside that sphere of ideal place with ideal weather.

- Keep expanding the sphere as far as comfortable, keeping the center of that sphere behind your navel.

- Take the time to enjoy the feeling inside and outside yourself—a feeling of lightness and ease, of peace and comfort. Feel like you are completely and absolutely accepted, appreciated, validated, and supported for who you really are. You have total permission to relax and be yourself. Feel the joy blooming out of your heart and spreading to the whole sphere around you.

- Slowly you are going to shrink the sphere by condensing and concentrating the feelings inside it. Make the sun shine brighter, the wind blow more softly, the grass appear greener, and keep condensing the sphere within you until it reaches the size of a small ball or a pearl spinning and spiraling behind your navel—a pearl made of pure condensed positive feelings.

- Be aware of the different loops of your Microcosmic Orbit and your different levels of individuation.

- Bring your pearl from behind your navel and make it spin and spiral at your navel, opening your power center and spreading all the positive feelings from your pearl there.

- Now, bring the pearl to your pelvic floor, spreading the good feelings there and attracting the positive feelings from the ground, from the Earth energy below you. Rest on this, absorbing the feelings of unconditional support. Bring the pearl to your sacrum and feel your sacrum opening to your life's momentum. Bring your pearl to your sexual center and feel the positive energy spreading there, awakening your sexual center to creativity and life enjoyment. Feel the wave of energy and your pearl circulating freely through the first loop of your Microcosmic Orbit.

- Bring your pearl to your Door of Life, stimulating it with the positive energy. Feel your life force being regenerated there, and then bring the pearl across to your navel where you feel your personal power very strongly, then down again to your sexual center and pelvic floor, then up your back to your sacrum and Door of Life.

- Bring your pearl up your back to your eleventh thoracic vertebra and feel it become more free and light, crossing over to your solar plexus where you find a regenerated sense of self.

- Let your pearl flow down your front and up your back and bring it up to your fourth thoracic vertebra, behind your heart, feeling the sense of freedom there, and cross over to your heart and feel it opening to more enthusiasm and high spirit.

- Let the pearl flow down your front and up your back, and bring it up to your seventh cervical vertebra, connecting with your ability to reach out and share. Let the enjoyable feelings spread from your pearl down your arms to your fingers, and cross over to your throat, spreading the positive feelings to your ability to verbalize, express, and speak from your heart.

- Let the pearl flow down your front and up your back to the base of your skull and let the base of your skull relax and open to the most positive dreams, crossing over to your mid-eyebrow, opening to a rich clarity of mind.

- Let your pearl flow down the front of your Microcosmic Orbit and up your back all the way to the top of your head, letting the positive feelings open your guiding center to the highest level of intuition, connecting inwardly to the pelvic floor and the Earth center through your Central Channel. Feel solidly anchored between heaven and earth, feel every energy center along your Microcosmic Orbit activated, breathing in and out the positive feelings from inside and out.

- Keep these feelings going as long as possible. Once in a while, during the day, try to capture the feeling of it again, and try to keep the momentum of this meditation going. It will get easier and easier with practice.

~~~~~~

... The song is to the singer, and comes back most to him,
The teaching is to the teacher, and comes back most to him,
The murder is to the murderer, and comes back most to him,
The theft is to the thief, and comes back most to him,
The love is to the lover, and comes back most to him,
The gift is to the giver, and comes back most to him—it cannot
    fail,
The oration is to the orator, the acting to the actor and actress,
    not to the audience,
And no man understands any greatness or goodness but his
    own, or the indication of his own ...

Walt Whitman, "A Song of the Rolling Earth"[12]

CHAPTER ★ 8

The Healing Practice

The Six Conditions for Healing

This chapter is directed toward Chi Nei Tsang practitioners, who are working with clients to heal the damage done over time, sometimes lifetimes, by mishandled energy charges. Chi Nei Tsang clients, too, will deepen their understanding of the process they are sharing with their practitioners.

Over the course of many years of practicing Chi Nei Tsang and helping clients process their emotional charges, and through my own healing experience, I have found that there are six fundamental conditions we have to fulfill in order to allow any given charge to heal completely. These conditions fall into a sequence and act as very straightforward steps, but they are not easy to take. In fact, they are probably the most difficult steps we can ever take. We are apt to take advantage of any opportunity presented to us to avoid them.

As explained in *Healing from Within*, these are the six conditions or sequence for healing, also called Surrendering to the Cycle of Healing, that are fulfilled during the healing process taking place within one or several Chi Nei Tsang sessions. These conditions are necessary to allow our guardian within to lower our defenses, to reverse the strategy from one of armoring, blind protection, hanging on to old familiar patterns, and stiffening, to one of change, transformation, and evolution. Figure 9 shows the conditions, juxtaposed to our universal symbol of the Five Elemental Forces of Nature.

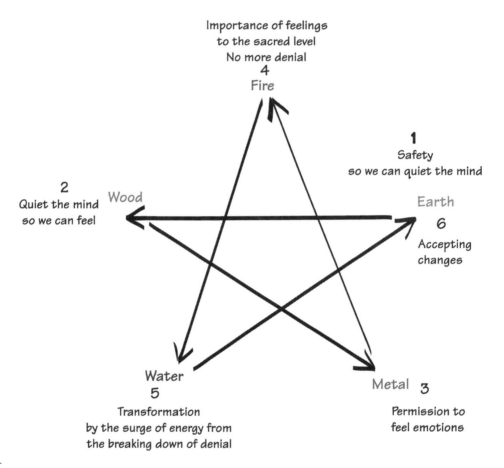

Surrendering to the cycle of healing

The six conditions for healing follow the cycle of surrendering,
which is the reverse of the control cycle

Importance of feelings
to the sacred level
No more denial
4
Fire

1
Safety
so we can quiet the mind

2
Quiet the mind
so we can feel   Wood

Earth
6
Accepting
changes

Water
5
Transformation
by the surge of energy from
the breaking down of denial

Metal 3

Permission to
feel emotions

Figure 9.
Surrendering to the
cycle of healing

Each condition falls into a sequence, and is the requisite for the next one.

1—We need to feel safe.

2—Our mind needs to quiet.

3—Our emotional self needs permission and support to feel.

4—All our feelings need to be recognized and validated to the highest degree of sacredness.

5—Our spirit needs to give us the green light for breakthrough and change.

6—We need to accept the changes and be supported and accepted while these changes are taking place.

These six conditions are described below, with a special focus on how practitioners can apply and monitor them during the Chi Nei Tsang healing process with clients.

1—We need to feel safe.

Safety is the first condition. Without this, the rational mind has to be switched on to look for a solution to the safety issue. This is the first checkpoint for our inner guide to make us aware that anything is wrong. There is no change possible if we don't know or don't feel what it is that we have to change. The power of denial, our ultimate protector from pain, keeps us unaware of an emotional charge if we lack the maturity, the support system, and the right time or place for its processing. We have to feel safe. So it is, therefore, important that the practitioner take all the steps necessary to make sure the clients feel so safe that they won't even need to think, which is the next condition for healing.

For many people, safety is about understanding, so do not hesitate to explain everything to them, down to the last detail if necessary. Education, by itself, is healing. Most people don't know what is going on with them. Many think that something is wrong when what they are actually experiencing is *awareness,* the first step of the healing process. Suppressing the symptoms will only make things worse. Giving them an explanation reassures them about the process. First, make them focus on everything they need to feel safe about what is going on before attempting to turn off their thinking process. The next step will be to prevent them from thinking.

The teaching role of the practitioner is extremely important. Many people won't understand the healing process at the strictly mental level. Educating them about it has to be done through example and entrainment, drawing them along with you. Most of the work in Chi-Kung and meditation is done to facilitate this crucial step in the healing process. These practices raise the energy of the practitioner in an evolutionary mode and tune it into the healing process, thus entraining the energy body of the client and supporting it in that direction. No amount of verbal explanation can replace the information relayed through energetic contact. The client literally needs to be submerged and cocooned in the practitioner's field of information. For this reason, the environment has to feel completely safe and the practitioner-client relationship must be extremely clear. Only then will the client's mind be able to quiet so that he or she can relax and allow emotions to come up.

To know that practitioners have experienced their own healing process through their training helps clients to feel safe during a healing session. Again, healing is about coaching someone else through something normal and natural that has been experienced by others time and time again. This is why it is a requirement for all practitioners-in-training to receive Chi Nei Tsang treatments before becoming certified. It is also why the most successful practitioners of Chi Nei Tsang are the ones who started studying it *after* they went through their own healing. They are the ones who attract clients without advertising. People "see" in them what they are looking for.

If you are a practitioner of any healing modality, no matter what you do, make sure that your client feels heard. Give feedback and systematically validate every feeling you get from that person. Also remember that some people just don't match with your own personality. They might not like you, or you might not like them. Sometimes gender, age, or even race can be a big issue. Don't take it personally. Remember that emotions cannot be reasoned with. Your clients might have already tried and failed. Their situation will change anyway, through the healing process. It is good, at least, to have that piece of awareness. Refer them to another practitioner with whom they might feel more comfortable. Also, sometimes the timing might not be quite right, but don't let this concern you. They'll come back when they are ready. They now know where to find you.

Please don't mold your approach into a standardized procedure to apply to every treatment. In healing, no one is standard, so standard procedures apply to no one. Adapt to the needs of each client. Some might need more explanation than others. Others don't want any explanations at all. You just need to give them extra support and appropriate help. Only experience can teach you to widen your expertise in approaching each client based on his or her specific needs.

The Chi-Kung exercises and meditations learned during the Chi Nei Tsang training—Space and Boundaries Chi-Kung, the Healing Buddha Palms, the Opening of the Microcosmic Orbit, and the Fusion of the Five Elemental Forces meditation—are invaluable for practitioners regardless of their healing modality to create a reassuring, personalized, empathic, and supportive presence during healing sessions.

2—Our mind needs to quiet.

The more we think, the less we feel. This is a prime characteristic of depression, when thinking tries to replace feeling. Our mind first needs to quiet to be able to listen and perceive before it can help our emotional self to feel more precisely during the next step in the healing process. The principle here is that we can't talk and listen at the same time. People who do so are the same people who talk to themselves all the time because they are emotionally hurt and afraid of feeling too much. They are also uncomfortable being in the present moment, which is the only place healing can happen. Thinking has to fade into the background for a while, leaving all the energy, space, and time to the expression of feelings.

When we quiet the mind, we allow more energy for emotional life. By the mind, I mean the rational, problem-solving, justifying, and judgmental mind, as opposed to the whole mind, which encompasses not only thinking but also feelings, intuition, practicality, and dreams. Problem solving is an important function of the rational mind, but unfortunately it has a tendency to stay switched on for many of us. Our rational mind turns everything into a problem to solve. But problem solving is actually quite easy to do, and if that were all there is to getting healthy, emotionally and mentally, then most forms of psychotherapy would be successful, immediate, and permanent.

The thinking process is necessary in establishing a relationship of confidence with the client. Once this has been accomplished, though, thinking needs to be switched off to allow the abstraction and irrationality of emotions to be witnessed without justification or judgment. The rational, critical, and judgmental aspects of the thinking process are usually what prevent us from being emotionally aware. With further training, though, the thinking process can change and actually help to deepen and refine the healing process. But first, clients learn to turn off the automatic reflexes of antagonism and judgment, to remain calm in the present moment, and to support the felt sense by unconditional acceptance—something well beyond conventional norms.

Remember, emotions are not rational. Emotions are not concerned with explanation or justification; this would be like asking for permission to feel, or, in the language of emotions, like asking for permission to live! The only thing emotions care about is validation, a testimony to their existence. Once this happens, our mind gives permission for our body to take over, and then moves out of the way. In all its innate intelligence, the body knows exactly what to do. It has to digest to allow us to outgrow emotional distress.

There is not enough energy in the body to think and feel intensely at the same time. This is one of the reasons why we dream when we sleep. Only during dreamtime can we be 100 percent emotional. This is why sometimes clients go into dreamtime during healing sessions. I have found that during sleep, the eyes follow the movements of the charges reflected in the movements of the intestines. To me, this means that there is a direct correlation between Rapid Eye Movement (REM) during sleep and intestinal motility because we dream about what we emotionally digest.

In short, no matter what comes up, practitioners should never be judgmental with clients. Most clients are already too judgmental with themselves. By turning off problem solving, justifying, and judgment, and tuning into the ability to feel, practitioners can train their clients to do the same with themselves, thus opening the doors of perception into the emotional realms.

3—Our emotional self needs permission and support to feel.

Once our mind quiets, more energy is available for feeling. Then emotions can really be felt for what they are, and for what they are not. They are neither thoughts that come into and go out of our mind, nor are they a matter of choice. Emotions are manifested in our body as a solid "substance," which I call a charge. This solid substance feels like it has a life of its own and moves around our body, creating imbalances in our metabolism and pressure in our head, joints, and back. Emotional charges do not just develop in our bodies the same way that thoughts or ideas do. Rather, they are more akin to contagions such as the common cold or sexually transmitted diseases, which spread through contact.

We are not responsible for the emotions we have. Our only responsibility is to be aware of them and manage them. It is difficult, however, to be responsible for this awareness and management when we are not taught how to do so. This is true especially when that "doing" *is not an active mental process*. Instead, it is our whole experience of the felt sense that happens at the core of our physical selves. A good example can be found in the notion of "forgiveness." When forgiveness is experienced only at the mental level, chances are that it is only spelling out denial, self-alienation, or at best, pure hypocrisy. Forgiveness is what happens to us when we outgrow and digest the grief and pain inflicted on us by others to the point that we are no longer negatively affected. Only then can we say that we have forgiven. Before this form of processing, though, forgiveness is only a good intention that hasn't yet had a chance to be manifested.

Forgiveness is actually mentally passive, and not something that we can mentally and actively manifest at will. This "passive" mental state is what has been called the Yin approach, or Yin perseverance in the Taoist tradition. Yin perseverance is about setting the right conditions, and then being flexible and trusting the process that the right result will come. Trusting involves a passive state of "stop and wait," with hope and faith in an intelligence and power higher than our own.

The goal for practitioners during this phase of emotional recognition and validation is to reflect to clients what they witness from the clients' body language and translate its emotional aspects. For this purpose, practitioners need to learn the emotional body language and to map out the meaning of emotional charges throughout the body. Every felt emotion has to be validated no matter how strange, uncomfortable, or wrong it might feel. The practitioner should always be supportive and validate *all feelings,* no matter what. There is always a good reason why we feel something, or we wouldn't feel it. However, the reason is not important. There is no such thing as "I shouldn't feel that way"—because we would never feel that way without reason. There is no need for justifying, either. Needing to justify an emotion, giving ourselves "a reason," or mental approval, is a judgmental attitude of mental arrogance that splits and binds the mental image of self against its emotional counterpart. This is crazy-making indeed!

For clients, this condition means that, instead of analyzing everything or trying to understand and interpret everything, our mind can be educated to validate things that are still incomprehensible. What is most important is to feel our undigested emotional charges so that we have no other option than to finally recognize and validate them, process them, digest them, and outgrow them.

4—All our feelings need to be recognized and validated to the highest degree of sacredness.

This is the place where many practitioners tend to get stuck. Once contact is made with the emotional charge, the client's old protective reflexes will try all at once to reverse the process by coming back to thinking and understanding. Don't let this happen. No more explanation is needed. We have already successfully gone through this process, or we wouldn't be here now. Don't re-trigger the client's thinking process! Keep the client in touch with the abstraction of the emotional charge. At this point, both of you can literally witness pain moving from the physical level to the emotional level. Get your client to focus on the familiarity of the feeling rather than on the explanation or, even worse, the justification. It doesn't matter why. What does matter is the feeling itself and having the client stay with it right here, right now, in this place and time of the present moment, where healing happens and time ceases to exist.

We now have to be careful not to minimize any feelings. This would provide clients with the ultimate escape from the entire healing process. At this point, when hidden feelings are revealed or rediscovered, when there is finally awareness about the quality, intensity, and number of feelings that were previously concealed, their soul is touched to the very core, that aspect of the deep self which is rarely accessed in everyday life. The felt sense of the soul comes into awareness as it changes, as opportunities arise to eliminate old feelings, to shed them like an old skin, never to be used again. Such a moment is as important and as sacred as a birth or death; indeed, it is both at the same time. The clients are leaving behind a part of themselves never to be seen again as they become renewed and more mature through the healing process. A page of their life has been turned, and they are beginning a new chapter. This is history in the making, a truly important and sacred moment.

5—Our spirit needs to give us the green light for breakthrough and change.

In every case of spontaneous healing, the most spectacular phase is that moment when a rush of energy comes, awakens the patient from his or her torpor, and reverses the ailment, often with a vigorous emotional outburst that seems impossible given the apparent weakness of the patient. Where is this energy coming from? In the old tradition, we were led to believe that it was coming from the healer, God, Satan, or some other external force. In reality, the energy is coming from the person, who has been conditioned to hold unconscious tensions that require tremendous amounts of energy to remain hidden. Think of the energy required to build, nourish, and protect a tumor from the immune system. How much energy has to be spent to prevent someone from breathing in certain places, to be out of alignment, to contract to the point of spasm and atrophy?

Once the protection is dropped, the spirit is freed, and the tensions holding the emotional charges are no longer needed. The layer of denial that was protecting the client from emotional pain collapses like a dam, and behind it comes the wave of energy that was used to hold the pattern of tension and the pathological factor in place. All that energy spent holding misalignments, chronic pain, tumors, rashes, and internal pressure is dislodged and recycles itself into that healing force that reinstates health. This is true healing energy unleashed, and it is irreversible. This is the transformational stage.

This stage is often spectacular, and can even be rather frightening for an inexperienced practitioner. Clients' reactions are unpredictable when confronted with what they have been trying so hard to hide from themselves. We have to have a lot of respect for our denial system. Our mind has to adapt our sense of reality around it, and when the truth comes out, our sense of reality is shattered, often causing a violent reaction of protest. Practitioners need to be prepared to restrain their clients in order to protect them from injury. Sometimes during the reaction, the client appears to be possessed and enduring some kind of wild and fearful exorcism. I have seen people jump off the massage table headfirst in one spastic contraction! But I have never encountered a situation where I felt at risk of being hurt, even during the worst of psychotic outbursts, at the peak of furor, with expression of murderous hatred and fists or feet striking table, floor, and walls. Practitioners have to remember that clients *are* conscious; they are witnessing their own catharsis, and a certain amount of control is always present. The danger arises when we are not aware of how much charge we have stored. That's what makes us do things we always thought we couldn't do. Once we go through the healing process, our awareness emerges, and we can feel worse than ever because we are now more aware! Paradoxically, even though it might not seem so, we are in much more control when we feel than when we are in total denial and experience that cold, insensitive urge that can make us commit the most atrocious acts of hatred. If you yourself have ever been through such an episode, you know that the tendency is to hurt yourself rather than others. Remember, also, that the main reason we are able to let ourselves go through such catharsis is because we trust, and have confidence, and feel safe and supported by the practitioner and the situation. This is, in fact, a privileged moment. Such a catharsis is easier to stop or prevent than to allow full expression. It is just following the natural urge brought on by the sudden freeing of trapped energy.

Sometimes clients can be completely catatonic, and appear to be paralyzed in a particular body stance or expression. Such paralysis can be expressed during the client's apparent sleep and manifest for a long time (perhaps up to two hours). Quite often, catharsis is manifested during such a deep sleep that clients can stop breathing for so long that their lips start to turn blue. This can be unsettling for practitioners and they might be tempted to interrupt the session. Remember though, that the main danger is the interruption of such a healing process. Whatever clients don't release now in the safety of the treatment room will have to be released later, often in series of nightmares, and it could take years to accomplish the same result that is achieved in the healing session.

Our mind is there to protect us from feeling bad. It has been well trained, twenty-four hours a day, for a long time, to prevent us from feeling something. If our spirit finally gives us the green light to feel that charge again, something that we promised ourselves a long time ago never to feel again, we can assume that the safety margin is huge. Only then can our spirit, our inner guide or guardian, give us the green light for the physical tensions to dissolve and liberate the energy needed for transformation. At this point, there is no turning back, for change is already taking place.

Note to Practitioners: Be aware of "fake" emotional releases. Such emotional outbursts come as a *reaction* to rather than as a *sensitivity* to emotions. Be careful of too much drama. Make sure that you are able to differentiate emotional sensitivity from emotional reaction. This is easy to recognize, as a reaction will repeat itself when the client is put in the same situation and reaches that stage of the treatment. A real emotional release *never* repeats itself—it releases only once, and for good. The "fake" release happens when clients are emotionally reactive rather than sensitive and never really allow themselves to feel completely. They merely react to the *thought* of emoting. It is then necessary to bring them back to the here and now, and make them experience and visualize, at the same time, the part of themselves that wants to heal and the part of themselves that is afraid of going through the suffering of the healing process and the changes involved. Make them breathe deeply while holding this visualization right in front of them, and proceed with the treatment.

Possible reactions you might encounter during the transformational stage include:

- Sudden deep sleep while working on the place where the person holds an emotional charge, evidenced by deep breathing, often loud snoring, and rapid eye movement signaling intense dream state.
- Deep sleep with spasms and sleep talking.
- Catatonic state.
- Hyperventilation with spasms in the extremities.
- Involuntary movements.
- Crying.
- Screaming.
- Cathartic and exorcism-like behavior.
- Tetany of the extremities and spasm of the facial muscles, sometimes from one-half hour to two hours.

6 — We need to accept the changes and be supported and accepted while these changes are taking place.

At this level, transformation is complete and healing has happened. There is no turning back; there is no reason for the old symptoms to ever reappear. However, sometimes the changes are drastic and not easy to accept. The client is in a very tired, fragile, and vulnerable state, very open to discouragement and the nocebo effect (the psychological response directly opposite to placebo—placebo heals, nocebo kills). Sometimes, just an innocent joke from a family member or a friend, or a doubting reaction from a doctor or other authority figure, can have a devastating impact at this stage of healing and could lead to catastrophe. I had one case where, even though all tumors and symptoms of cancer had disappeared, the client fell into a coma following a visit to her doctor and died a few days later. It is important to note that her husband had also just left her. Clients who are in the healing process should remain in a very supportive environment until they are mentally strong enough to hold the changes on their own. They should be careful and take time for recovery to allow the changes to "sink in," to integrate them. Some time away, such as a retreat in a pleasant setting, is always a good idea. Just make sure that the client is not thrown into a bad emotional setting after healing has taken place.

Global Body Attitude and Holism

The Three Musketeers of Healing

When addressing health, there are three primary approaches or perspectives possible:

- The metabolic approach, using internal medicine.
- The structural approach, working with the alignment of the body.
- The emotional and mental approach, using psychotherapy.

Figure 10. Global body attitude and the three musketeers of therapeutic approaches (right)

Global Body Attitude
and
The Three Musketeers of Therapeutic Approaches

The three approaches possible to treat any illness are either the metabolic approach, in case of internal problems;the structural approach, in case of pain resulting from external or internal misalignment;and emotional approach for all mental symptoms and psychosomatic responses. These are the "Three Musketeers". But there is the fourth character, D'Artagnan. who is in fact the hero without whom there is no story possible. D'Artagnan is Chi:the power of life, the energy that uplifts the spirit, that has to be added to all modalities in order to make them healing. Each modality, when using Chi, can greatly help people in their healing process, but only Chi Nei Tsang actively and simultaneously uses the three different approaches with the added Chi of the applied Chi-Kung from the practitioners and the active meditations (Chi-Kung) taught to the clients.

Internal medicine
Surgery
Pharmacopea
Drugs
Herbs
Nutrition
Chi-Kung
Meditation
Reiki
Chi Nei Tsang

Any change, whether in our metabolism, the structure of our body or in our emotions, has a direct influence on the way we breathe, and the way we breathe directly inflences our metabolism,our moods, and our structure. Changing our breath changes our energy, changing our energy changes our breath. Breath generates Chi. Breath is the motor and generator, Chi is the information and energy produced.

Metabolism

Any change and shift in the structure of the body, either external (spine, rib cage, hips, shoulders, feet, head) or internal (diaphragm, weight distribution shift of the intestines) has a direct effect on the functions of the internal organs and the balance of the metabolism.

There is no question that feeling upset in our metabolic system makes us feel emotionally upset, and feeling healthy makes it easier to be in a good mood.

Any positive change in the metabolism such as detoxifying the liver and kidneys, balancing the digestion, clearing the intestinal tract, equili--brating blood pressure, reversing from a chronic stressful sympathetic response to a more healing parasympathetic mode, inhibiting the production of stress hormones such as adrenaline and insuline, has a positive impact on the structure of the body.

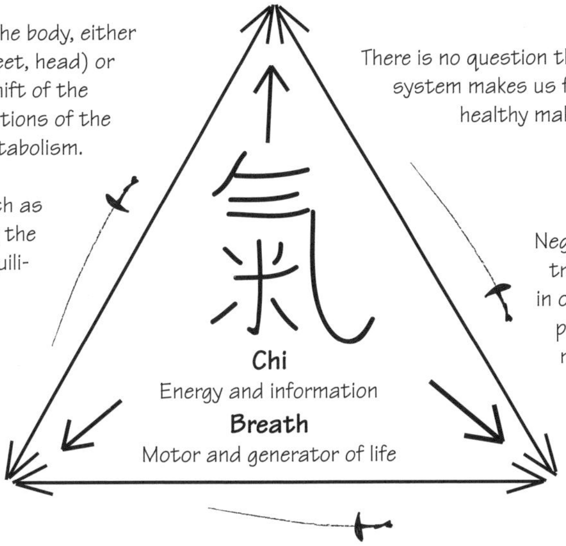

Negative emotions and bad feelings translate as stress and pressure in our internal organs, raising blood pressure, interfering with cardiac rhythm, inhibiting the production of digestive juices and enzymes, and restricting breath.

Structure

Chi Nei Tsang
Chi-Kung
Feldenkrais
Shiatsu
Massage and body work
Dance
Yoga
Pilates
Physical therapy
Chiropractics
Surgery

There is a natural tendency to hold ourselves diferently according to the way we feel. The structural body attitude reflects our emotional attitude (holding our shoulders high and rounded when feeling overburdened) and holding our structure in a certain way influences the way we feel and think (frowning or rounding our back when we feel upset).

Emotions

Chi Nei Tsang
Meditation
Psychotherapy
Chi-Kung
Massage and body work
Reiki
Arts
Theatre
Music
Dance
Crafts

**Global Body Attitude
Holistic Physiological Summary**

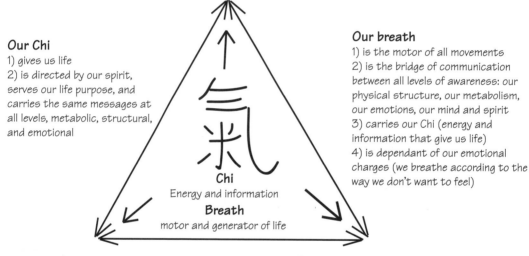

Our viscera
1) not only digest our food but
also has to digest our emotions
2) is the first system being affected
by emotional charges via our
Enteric Nervous System
3) holds and stores emotional charges
according to their meaning, history,
and state of digestion
4) will digest emotional charges only
when given permission (felt)

Our Chi
1) gives us life
2) is directed by our spirit,
serves our life purpose, and
carries the same messages at
all levels, metabolic, structural,
and emotional

Our breath
1) is the motor of all movements
2) is the bridge of communication
between all levels of awareness: our
physical structure, our metabolism,
our emotions, our mind and spirit
3) carries our Chi (energy and
information that give us life)
4) is dependant of our emotional
charges (we breathe according to the
way we don't want to feel)

Chi
Energy and information
Breath
motor and generator of life

Our physical structure and its alignment
1) holds our weight and balance the safest and
most economical way according to what we don't
want to feel
2) takes a tremendous amount of energy to be
out of alignment (invests against emotional pain)
3) reflects perfectly our mental and emotional
states

Our emotional charges
1) rules our breath
2) needs to be digested
3) are digested only when permission is given by our
higher self (spirit) to feel them
4) when undigested, are held in significant parts of
the body at the structural level, affecting function,
range of motion, coordination; and stored at the vis-
-ceral level, affecting metabolic and mental processes

Figure 11.
Global body attitude
and the holistic
physiological
summary

When these three approaches are used in one modality, it is called a holistic modality. I equate this with Alexandre Dumas' three musketeers of legendary fame (see Figures 10 and 11). I use French literature to illustrate my understanding of healing methods because I have found a great similarity in the way Alexandre Dumas uses his main characters to tell stories. Even though the title of the book is *The Three Musketeers*, for Athos, Portos, and Aramis, the real hero is Dartagnan, a young cadet of the seventeenth-century French royal officers' academy, who is not even a musketeer. While the different episodes and stories involve either one, two, or three of the musketeers, Dartagnan is *always* present. Without him, there would be no story. Most of the episodes successfully conclude with the intervention of all the heroes with their *cris de ralliement: "Tous pour un et un pour tous!"*—"All for one and one for all!" This summarizes, for me, a true holistic approach.

In terms of healing, especially in Chi Nei Tsang, the single most important factor is Chi: the nonviolent energy containing the right information—Dartagnan. No Dartagnan, no story; no Chi, no Chi Nei Tsang! From the metabolic perspective of internal medicine (the first musketeer), herbs, nutrition, or Chi-Kung can address the quality of energy and the information particular to each case. Remember, there is no such thing as a standard procedure. A standard procedure would only apply to a standard person, and I have never met one. To address authentic individuals, Chi has to be used.

The same applies to the structural approach to healing (the second musketeer). Physical therapy, chiropractics, podiatry, orthodontics, massage therapy, and many other types of bodywork do not address the personality and quality of Chi, the intelligence of the body, and the reason why we decide to invest so much time and energy into a physical behavior that creates pain. If Chi is not used to address the pattern of tension, no healing is possible.

Psychotherapy (the third musketeer) plays an important role in bringing awareness to mental and emotional distress—an indispensable step in healing. However, when touch is systematically avoided, and thinking is used to understand, justify, and correct feelings as an attempt to change behavior, it is no wonder that the healing process can take such a long time! From a Taoist perspective, healing through thinking would be just impossible. Thinking cannot control emotions because Wood cannot cut Metal; only Metal can cut Wood. From a true holistic perspective, addressing mental and emotional distress without touching the body is distant healing. It would be like trying to fix a TV monitor with a remote control. Distant healing works, but it does require power and special skills to make and maintain contact. Healing without contact is just impossible.

In a true holistic approach, the three perspectives of metabolism, structure, and emotions are systematically addressed. This is extremely rare. Most dentists don't treat tooth decay by addressing metabolic imbalance or stress level, orthodontists don't usually address the alignment of the vertebrae when fitting braces, and medical doctors usually don't address the emotional life of their clients before prescribing drugs or surgery. When such practitioners refer to themselves as "holistic," it usually boils down to referring patients to a vast array of health care practitioners (surgeons, dentists, chiropractors, massage therapists, psychotherapists) who have no real common denominator. Far from unifying our individual health care and looking at it as a "whole"—as in holistic—such an attitude actually increases the fragmentation of the health care system, and winds up costing us more without addressing a true healing process.

Chi is the linking factor between the three primary approaches to health care, and it is the indispensable ingredient for any true holistic healing modality. Chi manifests through the firm intention to promote life, health, and well-being (see Figure 1 on p. 16 and Figure 12 on p. 151).

To my knowledge, only practitioners of Chi Nei Tsang, a few practitioners of pre-Cultural Revolution Traditional Chinese Medicine, and few practitioners of modalities derived from traditional non-allopathic healing modalities—Feldenkrais, Reiki, Traeger, and Breema, for example—use a true holistic approach, addressing Chi in their practices. All others can't help but follow the conditioning of their upbringing by trying to fix, repair, or correct. Even though I refer many clients to practitioners of other modalities, I never send a client to surgery, or a chiropractic adjustment, for example, without having addressed the emotional charge behind the symptoms. For a greater chance of a successful outcome, we get rid of the emotional charges behind the need for chiropractic adjustment or surgery. When a client is in need of orthodontics or teeth implants, I make sure that we do a whole course of Spino-Mandibular Equilibration[14] or Cranio-Sacral work. This will ensure that the dental intervention is not going to interfere with the proper movement of the bones of the skull or the mobilization of the spine, pelvis, legs, and feet.

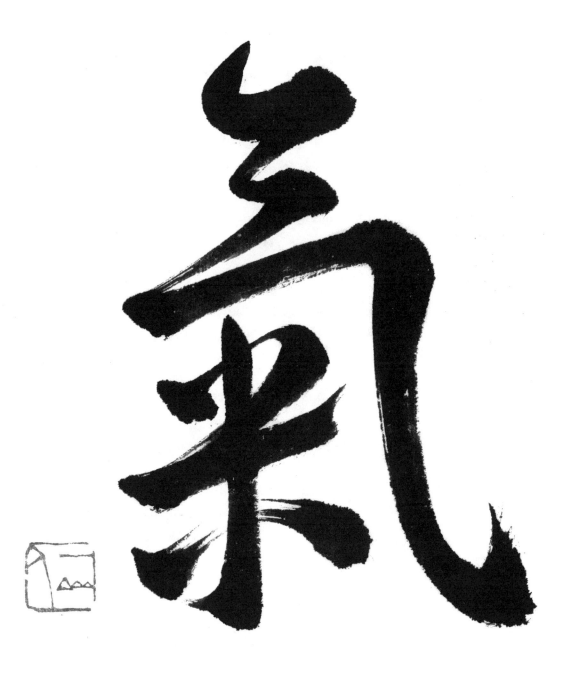

Chi, the breath of life.
Chi is the indispensable ingredient for any true holistic healing modality
and manifests through the firm intention to promote life, health, and well-being.

Figure 12.
Chi, the
breath of life

Case Study: Jane

Let's look at a hypothetical case, a composite of different actual occurrences often found in the same person.

Jane has painful scoliosis with a right anterior intercostal pain with nausea and migraine headaches on the right side of the head and pronounced gum recession on the right side of the mouth, all accompanied by frequent nightmares and insomnia.

- Typically, an internist will prescribe pills for the headache, other pills for insomnia, surgical removal of the gallbladder for gallstones, and send Jane to a dentist for the gums, to a chiropractor for the back pain, and to a psychotherapist for the nightmares.
- A chiropractor might temporarily alleviate her back pain through osseous adjustments, prescribe a gallbladder flush for her gallstones, send Jane to a dentist for the gum recession, and prescribe yoga or meditation classes for insomnia.
- A dentist might do a deep cleaning and disinfecting of her gums, send Jane to a naturopath to address a suspected gallbladder problem, and to a chiropractor or massage therapist for her back pain.
- A psychotherapist might help her uncover deeply hidden emotional charges that provoke bad posture, and might be able to have Jane come to terms with an old issue of chronic fits of anger inherited from a family pattern. He or she would probably send Jane to an internist for her intercostals pain and to a dentist for her gum recession.

All of these health care practitioners will address the specific symptoms as problems to fix and send Jane to a different specialist for anything they themselves don't treat. Nevertheless, none of these different treatments will really help her to heal by connecting the different symptoms into one pattern or tendency of the body, which has a deep meaning to be addressed. All of the health care practitioners involved are using a different healing musketeer, but Dartagnan is nowhere to be seen.

If Jane shows up for a Chi Nei Tsang treatment, all three approaches will be addressed. There is no need for the Chi Nei Tsang practitioner to attempt to address any symptom or "fix" anything because the use of Chi (Dartagnan) will naturally trigger the inner healing response, not only by connecting all of the symptoms, but also by addressing the root of each of Jane's symptoms.

In a Chi Nei Tsang treatment, we would:

- First, make Jane expand her breath and progressively guide her to breathe where it is not easy for her to breathe on her own.
- Second, manually coach her colon to ease its pull on the diaphragm and to promote a deeper breath.
- Laterally open the right side of her rib cage through guided breath and light touch, to release the gallbladder and promote the flow of bile.
- Expand her breath to the right side of Jane's rib cage and apply the Peace Touch method (see Chapter 9) to connect her with the emotional charges stored there, to promote their mental recognition and transit, as well as to release the tension in her gallbladder and bile duct where gallstones are trapped.
- If the right conditions are met, Jane might very well release the whole pattern of tension that makes her hold the right side of her rib cage tight, provoking scoliosis, and causing the tension in her neck, shoulders, and jaws with a restriction of the blood flow to her brain. This is a common holding pattern that causes headaches.
- Finally, Spino-Mandibular Equilibration, Cranial-Sacral Therapy, and/or some Feldenkrais sessions might be necessary and beneficial to teach her nervous system to maintain the new alignment resulting from the shift in her consciousness.

A scenario like Jane's is not uncommon in my practice. I regularly get gallbladder complaints, often from people who have already had their gallbladder surgically removed but still experience pain. Such experience has taught me that the pain does not come from a gallstone but from a nervous spasm of the bile duct and the surrounding tissues. When the spasm is dealt with, gallstones are naturally, safely, and painlessly evacuated. When the body gets through the crisis, it is ready to release the charge that prevents the gallbladder from functioning properly. Physiologically, the gallbladder takes the overflow from the liver.

This is also true for the emotional aspect of the gallbladder. Gallstones can be considered a psychosomatic response to prolonged emotional stress. As an attempt to hide the charge and to protect the individual from suffering at the emotional level, the body will twist and contract in a pattern of tension to cover the gallbladder area, provoking scoliosis and chronic contractions in the right shoulder and neck with habitual jaw clenching and, often, teeth grinding at night.

The Four Stages of the Healing Process

Four stages happen during the Chi Nei Tsang healing process: awareness (pain), confusion (resistance), breakthrough (transformation), and, finally, surrender (acceptance). Let's look at them, one by one.

Awareness

Awareness is the first stage of the healing process. It is the figurative doormat. Some of us can stand on this doormat forever without ever opening the door or entering the healing process at all. This is the stage of symptoms. Something within us is letting us know that something is wrong and that it needs attention. So we experience pain. The longer we stand on the doormat, the more chronic the symptoms become, and the more used to them we get, the more we identify with them. Awareness requires power. Awareness is the flag our guardian spirit waves at us to let us know that we now know better, that we now are more mature, we now have more strength, support, and life experience to address something that we couldn't before. It takes strength to be sensitive. It takes a lot of power to know what we do that puts and keeps us in misery.

Once clients enter my office, I know that they have already done a good percentage of the work. They already have the awareness that something has to change, and they have the maturity and the support system to allow them to seek help. They have already started their healing process.

Confusion

There is no healing without confusion. Confusion and hesitation always come as a resistance to change. Everyone wants to heal, but no one wants to change! Confusion is what happens when we realize that the map we have been following up to now is outdated. The sense of security the map provided was an illusion attached to a feeling of familiarity we had with it. So we decide to throw the map out the window, and now we really feel lost! But the longer we remain lost in this unfamiliar territory, the more confused we become about what direction to take. Thus, the more we have to explore, the more accurate the new map is going to be. This is the difficult stage of being caught between a very uncomfortable yet familiar place where we always get hurt, and a more comfortable yet unfamiliar place, which makes us face the fear of the unknown. Entering the healing process is like walking through a curved tunnel—we don't know where the end is. It could be around the next bend! The question is, how long will it take to get through the tunnel?

Healing only happens in the present, and the present is eternity! This is the time to use our rational mind to remind us that, no matter what, there is no turning back. We have to keep moving forward. We have to be flexible and use Yin perseverance to get us through this. The longer we stay confused, the better and more accurate our new map will be.

Breakthrough

Paradoxically, once we allow ourselves to be completely lost in the eternity of the present moment, then breakthrough happens. Suddenly, here we are, knowing that there is no turning back. A part of us will never be seen again because we have changed! The new information we gained from the tedious exploration of the previous stage of confusion has paid off—we have successfully integrated the new information. We know better, and our body reacts differently. We feel different, and even think differently. We have outgrown ourselves and achieved victory! Naturally, we might have some residual scars, but we survived, and there is no way that we will ever again be affected by the same symptoms.

Surrender

Change also has its particular problems. We are no longer the same to ourselves, and we are no longer the same to others. We are no longer who we are expected to be. This can cause trouble in relationships with family, friends, and co-workers. It is not unusual for divorce, career change, and relocation to follow the healing phase of transformation.

Since there is no turning back, we have to surrender to the forces of change and evolution. Hanging on to the past is no longer an option. Healing has already happened, and change is taking place. We are different now, so in order not to manifest the conditions again that brought on the original sickness, we have to accept the change!

Virtues and Flaws of Practitioners

The Five Virtues: Practicality, Sensitivity, Will, Mind, and Spirit

Five virtues characterize Chi Nei Tsang practitioners, and each is linked to one of the Five Elemental Forces of Nature.

Practicality (Earth): In Chi Nei Tsang, we believe that the primary virtue of practitioners is to carry the power of their Chi-Kung in their treatments, to be able to apply the supportive energy of the Five Elemental Forces of Nature, starting with the Earth attributes of unconditional support, validation, adaptation, nurturing, and comfort. Earth is the central element that holds the present moment where healing happens. In many traditions, people regularly pray to Earth deities and spirits for their healing. The traditional representation of the healing Earth "Spirit" is usually a feminine figure often found in a grotto near a natural spring, as in Our Lady of Lourdes, a famous pilgrimage site in southern France where many spontaneous recoveries have been reported. This is a good way to connect with the Earth force and healing. Earth is central and immediate, here and now. Because healing happens in the present, practitioners should always start by connecting with Earth and bringing the treatment to the here and now, connecting with the practical thing to do for this particular person at this particular time and place.

Sensitivity (Metal): Next comes connecting with feelings through the breath by opening to the Metal elemental force and its attributes of sensitivity, caring, and sharp but nonjudgmental way of cutting right through things in a very cool way. The Metal attitude is one of pure reflection, like a mirror reflecting the impressions and physical expressions during treatments. It is the ability to be emotionally very sensitive, and yet very precise and without mercy in terms of bringing everything into clarity and out of hiding. A good practitioner can use humor (Fire controls Metal) to temper the sharpness of the emotional sensitivity during the treatment, but should always stay sharp and never compromise.

Will (Water): Water virtue is about fluidity, great flexibility, attention, and creativity in the treatment. The practitioner should never be afraid to innovate. Every treatment is a new treatment, every client is different, and the practitioner needs to adapt every technique to the new situation. What is important is not the technique, but rather the healing principles that the techniques need to bring about. Water is also the power of regeneration, creation, and cleansing—the power of life itself. Practitioners need to absorb Water energy in order to bring its attributes to their treatments.

Mind (Wood): Practitioners need to quiet their own mind to help calm their clients into the nonrational realm of the healing response. At the same time, however, they need to stay focused on bringing clients to the next step of evolution and holding the space (Wood controls Earth) so that clients continue to feel safe. It is important that practitioners know their art so they can answer any question without hesitation. This will help clients feel safe and remain in the healing mode.

Spirit (Fire): In Traditional Chinese Medicine, the concept of Spirit (Shen) is a very important one. The first thing that Chinese physicians do before accepting anyone as a client is to look in the person's eyes. If they see spirit, they might accept that person as a client. But if they see no spirit, they will refuse. No matter how benign the symptoms, they know that it might take forever to improve, if at all, and they don't want to risk their reputation by treating someone who cannot get well.

Practitioners have to keep their spirit high to have guidance and to connect their clients with their own spirit. This is done by example and entrainment. This is one important reason practitioners have to practice their Chi-Kung and meditations regularly.

Note to Practitioners: You have to be an open conduit for the clear transmission of the Five Elemental Forces of Nature, the power of growth, the power of healing, and the evolution of human consciousness. You need to keep your spirit high so that the Chi flows from you toward your clients instead of the reverse. If your spirit is lower than your clients', you'll be loading up with their releases. Ground the treatment and run your Chi-Kung (Microcosmic Orbit, Healing Buddha Palms, Fusion) so that the energy by-products from treatment either get grounded or re-cycled. Also, when you raise your spirit, it makes it easier for your clients to do the same and recover faster. To be in touch with your spirit is to be in touch with your life purpose. The main reason we get sick is from be-ing out of touch, from having fallen away from our "Way," our Tao.

The Five Character Flaws:
Recklessness, Timidity, Short Temper, Self-Importance, and Excessive Concern About Appearances

In *The Art of War,* of ancient legendary Taoist fame, Sun Tzu describes the five character flaws of the warrior: recklessness, timidity, short temper, self-importance, and excessive concern about appearances. These flaws can undoubtedly be applied to peace warriors and healers alike. To help you better understand how, I will explain these flaws as they applied to the early years of my healing practice.

Recklessness: When I was studying Chi Nei Tsang with Master Chia, I couldn't wait to go home and try the techniques I had learned on my clients. For each technique, I would make a list of clients on whom I knew it would work beautifully. Unfortunately, in my haste to apply techniques, I lost all sense of practicality. Even though my mind was focused on the goal, I was out of sync with the current needs of my clients. This characterizes a major Earth weakness of being nonsup-portive of the client with too much planning and lack of appreciation for what is going on in the present (Wood overcontrolling Earth).

Timidity: Humbled by my recklessness, I did a 180-degree turn and became timid with my treatments, losing perspective again, and un-consciously withdrawing the mental and emotional support that my clients so desperately needed. This is again a major Earth weakness compounded by a weak Fire, resulting in low spirit.

Short temper: I then started to blame the poor results on the "laziness" of my clients and gave them too much homework. Here, the Fire imbalance of impatience controls the sensitivity of Metal.

Self-importance: I couldn't believe that I, who practiced so much, knew so much, and was one of the best practitioners alive, could be the cause of failure in my treatments. This caused me to distance myself further from these early clients of mine, and of course, they never came back.

Excessive concerns about appearances: Losing clients didn't look good, but I had enough sense not to give up. I kept practicing, and eventually became aware of what I was doing and was able to evolve and change. It took a long time. If I had had too many concerns about the way things looked for me, I would have given up, my healing spirit would have plummeted, and with it all my connections to the elemental forces. All would have been lost!

CHAPTER ☆ 9

Touching and Being "in Touch"

The Healing Touch Versus the Fixing Touch

This chapter, too, speaks primarily to Chi Nei Tsang practitioners. But clients, or potential clients, can certainly benefit from the guidelines here.

As soon as our touch carries the message of "fixing" or correcting something, it conveys the emotional message that whatever is being touched is "wrong" or "in need of repair." Remember that every part of the human body is human; therefore, it will react as humanly as we would in the same situation. When we are made to feel wrong, our first reflexes are understandably protest, defense, and denial. We are not intentionally wrong just for the sake of being wrong. The worst reaction can always be justified by lack of information, misinterpretation, misguidance, fear, or other negative emotions, and generally comes out of the best of intentions, which is the intention of "fixing." We have to understand that there is no such thing as a "wrong" emotion. As far as the emotional self is concerned, there is no need to fix because there is nothing broken. Generally, the body is trying to do the best it can with a painful situation. Correction would add insult to injury.

In fact, any reaction from "negative" emotions will automatically create a chain reaction leading to poor behavior. To deal with the emotional response of any part of ourselves, we need to address it the same way we ought to address the emotions of infants and children (or any living being, for that matter)—validating the emotions instead of ignoring, minimizing, or contradicting them. I believe that the problems the modern world experiences in both education and relationship are because of its lack of emotional intelligence and its callousness when confronted with emotional responses.

The therapeutic or healing touch has to come from a place of unconditional support where there is no room for misinterpretation. Practitioners have to learn to be aware of their space and boundaries at the physical, mental, and emotional levels, to not create an adverse reaction in their clients. Awareness of our own space and boundaries also allows us to better perceive where these boundaries are in our clients. Practitioners need to integrate their Space and Boundaries Chi-Kung, as taught at the Chi Nei Tsang Institute, to provide safety through their touch. If their touch doesn't feel safe to their clients, practitioners have to touch through the clients' hands until safety is established. If we are seeking healing, we usually come from having suffered violence and we have already suffered very intrusive allopathic procedures and need to know mentally and emotionally that we won't be insulted again. The emotional body doesn't speak English, or French, or Mandarin. It speaks the universal language of feelings. Like a baby, the only language it speaks is smiling when happy and crying when uncomfortable, but it communicates very accurately through touch. When we are in emotional distress, a compassionate hug, a pat on the shoulder, or a caring hand-hold carries more information than long discourses. This is Chi at work.

The body is already designed to be addressed through a touch that provides no resistance and requires no effort from practitioners other than to learn to relax and open to the flow of Chi, with nonverbal communication. It is extremely simple but apparently very difficult to do because of the severity of conditioning and judgment about *touch*. Touching is generally considered taboo in this culture and mostly banned from psychotherapy. The banning of touch is understandable to prevent abuse and violence in a context of ignorance. However, in terms of therapy, in my opinion, there is no healing possible without touch. To be able to touch in the right way with absolute nonviolence is at the root of all teachings at the Chi Nei Tsang Institute. From beginning to graduation, after students have been trained in the highest practices of the Fusion of the Five Elemental Forces meditation, the Healing Buddha Palms Chi-Kung, and in Space and Boundaries Chi-Kung, the main training focuses on developing the ability to touch. Touching has to be done peacefully in such a way that clients don't feel the practitioner, but rather feel themselves. Practitioners learn to disappear behind their own touch to let clients discover themselves. This takes years to master and a lifetime to cultivate. It is a skill indispensable to the evolution and preservation of the human race.

The Power of Gentleness: The Power Touch, Listening Touch, and Peace Touch

Three types of gentle touching are utilized in Chi Nei Tsang healing sessions, as described below.

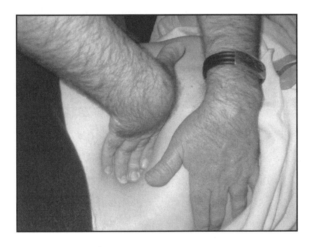

Figure 13.
The healing touch

Power Touch is the ability to touch powerfully with neither muscle tension nor threat. Nonviolence doesn't mean not using force; nonviolence means not abusing force. To make sure that the message of nonviolence is received, touch has to convey the least flexion possible, using mostly extensor muscles and extending the Chi. The hands and fingers never grab, and the fingers are in full extension, bending backward like a paintbrush (see Figure 13). The softer the fingers, the more deeply we are able to reach into the body without inflicting pain. By relaxing our shoulders and bending our fingers and hands backward like brush hairs all the way to the wrists, we accomplish several things:

- We send a message of nonaggression. Because we can't contract our fingers in this position, it feels like we could never hurt anyone.
- We have to wait until we are invited in, so we can't force our way and intrude.
- Even though we can't use muscular power in this position, we are structurally stronger.
- Because we wait and don't force, we can feel the quality and listen to the subtle movements of the tissues.
- Because this is done with gentleness, there is no limit to the amount of power that can be used this way.

This can only be fully understood through practice. It is an esoteric practice using the same power of martial arts such as Karate, Judo, and Aikido; it is the Way of the Empty Hand (Karate), the Way of Suppleness (Judo), and the Way of Harmony (Aikido).

Listening Touch is a firm and supportive touch that repeats everything that is felt by extending the Chi throughout the whole body with a gentle vibration or a gentle rocking. It is an active listening, which validates that the voice of the tissues is being heard throughout the entire person. Listening Touch is constantly asking the body, "Do you feel this? Are you saying that? Is that what you feel?" Using the rule of Yin perseverance, it follows with absolute flexibility, never correcting or directing. It is an emotionally supportive touch, as when listening to a friend tell you her problems, not expecting to be helped, but just asking to be heard and be emotionally validated.

Peace Touch is the next technical step to bring clients to the core of their being. Peace Touch is utilized to help clients connect with their core issues when they are unable to keep their awareness on the physical location of the emotional charge. It uses the fundamental Aikido concept of nonopposition of forces, blending and drawing the partner into a vacuum created by his or her own movement. It consists of applying Power Touch to make contact with the location where awareness has been withdrawn, and then creating a vacuum by withdrawing our Chi, while still maintaining physical contact. This vacuum literally draws the clients' breath and consciousness down to the area being touched, filling this space with their awareness. By maintaining the

Peace Touch, we create a space where clients feel safe and supported enough to be with their localized issues. Without Peace Touch, clients would most likely never be able to bring their awareness to this part of themselves on their own, and the emotional charges would remain trapped and undigested.

Case Study: The Body Is Stronger than Drugs

I had a client who, after recovering from an accident, was still in so much pain that he was contemplating suicide. He had taken all the painkillers possible. Doctors had succeeded at first, by numbing the pain or making him so dull that he put less focus on his suffering, but the pain was still there. Over time, he required larger and larger doses of drugs until he finally reached the point where he no longer experienced any relief. His body had outgrown the drugs. When I put my fingers on his back, using the gentlest of touches, the muscles started to relax and tensions melted away. After barely twenty minutes of a combination of Listening Touch and Peace Touch, he experienced the first relief from pain in eight months. That night he slept peacefully for the first time since his accident.

Healing Buddha Palms Chi-Kung

Healing Buddha Palms Chi-Kung is one of the most important exercises for practitioners of Chi Nei Tsang. It consists of actively connecting what we call the Three Fundamental Forces and the Personal Forces through our bones like antennas and feeding our Microcosmic Orbit and the rest of ourselves with it.

- Start with Earth Relationship Chi-Kung in a good standing position. Sink as you breathe in and push your weight into the ground as you breathe out. Your feet should be parallel and shoulder-width or hip-width apart. Let your feet relax and feel your weight sink into the ground.

- Smile into your feet and feel the ground smiling back at your feet, softening, becoming more comfortable. Feel your head to be suspended from the ceiling, the weight of your spine hanging from your head, and your hips hanging from your spine. Feel your joints loose, and let your body sway a little so you won't get stiff.

- Open the Seven Loops of Individuation, and then practice Opening the Microcosmic Orbit.

- Initiate Bone-Breathing (*Healing from Within,* p. 18) until you are aware of all your bones. Then practice Bone-Packing (*Healing from Within,* p. 68). Be aware of your bones working like antennas, connecting to the Fundamental Forces. If you don't know your Bone-Breathing or Bone-Packing yet, just be aware for now that your bones are the most crystallized part of your body. They work as antennas, picking up information flowing at the right frequency for you.

- Be aware of the rhythm of your Chi at your navel—the rhythm within your breath that feels like your heartbeat. Match this rhythm at the center of your palms, the bottoms of your feet, the top of your head, and your pelvic floor, setting the same frequency throughout your whole body.

- Raise your hands over your head, palms facing up, index fingers slightly stretched to open the palms. Mentally connect with all the information beyond human comprehension that we call Kosmic Energy. Absorb this Kosmic Energy through your palms, pack it inside your bones as you breathe in, and let it flow through the rest of your body as you breathe out.

- Lower your hands in front of your forehead, palms facing out. Mentally connect with the whole of the human universe with its laws, knowledge, and traditions we call Universal Energy. Absorb this Universal Energy through your palms, pack it inside your bones as you breathe in, and let it flow through the rest of your body as you breathe out.

- Bring your arms down, forearms and hands in front of your body at the height of the navel, palms facing down. Mentally connect with all the Earth attributes of nurturing, harmony, and unconditional support we call Earth Energy. Absorb Earth Energy through your palms, pack it inside your bones as you breathe in, and let it flow through the rest of your body as you breathe out.

- Drop your thumbs (palms down), bend your elbows and pull your arms back, aligning the "Tiger Mouth" or acupuncture point LI-4 (the fleshy web on the back of your hand between your thumb and index finger) of each hand with the "eye" of each hip. Feel the energy passing between the Tiger Mouth points through the hips and abdomen.

- Feel solidly anchored between heaven and earth.

- Connect with the first loop of your Microcosmic Orbit—the pelvic floor, sacrum, and sexual center—for establishing foundations of support (see Chapter 5).

- Holding the same position of the arms, with your palms facing up, turn your fingertips to the eye of your hips.

- Holding the same position of the arms, with your palms facing up, turn your fingers pointing forward, aligning the "Chi knife" side of the hands with the eye of your hips.

- Release your elbows, bring your forearms in front of you with palms facing up. Relax your shoulders, connect to your personal source of power, your spiritual Chi—whatever feeds your spirit, whatever you like most in life, whatever gives you enthusiasm (such as your favorite people, animals, geographical location, weather, trees, color, stars, rhythm, or a piece of music). Pack this inside your bones as you breathe in, and let it flow through the rest of your body as you breathe out.

- Turn your wrists so your palms are facing down, forearms and hands at the height of the navel, connecting with the ground right here and now. Connect with Earth Chi, the present moment, whatever allows you to be right here right now, your entire support system, including your ancestors. Feel that support under your feet and in the palms of your hands and pack it inside your bones as you breathe in, and let it flow through the rest of your body as you breathe out.

- Keep connecting with your support system and the Earth Chi, your spiritual Chi, and the Kosmic, Universal, and Earth forces, while bringing both of your palms over your navel and connecting with your inner Chi there. Be aware of this energy and information circulating through all the levels of your Microcosmic Orbit.

Now, rest. You deserve it.

Conclusion—Healing, Critical Mass, and the Evolution of Human Consciousness

Why is it so difficult to meditate, to pray, to do Chi-Kung, yoga, dance, exercise, and other activities that would make our life so much better? Because, unfortunately, such practices are not common enough. And yet, it is so easy to waste time in front of the TV screen or a video game, even when we don't really feel like it, because it is so common to so many people. It is a problem of critical mass. Every time someone gathers the courage to change and go through the healing process, every time someone decides to meditate with the sincere intention to grow as a person, to improve, and to outgrow his or her condition, it makes it easier for anyone else to do so. The time has come when meditation and Chi-Kung need to be part of everyday life, like some form of internal hygiene. Once the number of people practicing reaches a certain number, attaining and surpassing the critical mass, it will feel natural to anyone and become an ordinary event like taking meals at regular times, attending to personal hygiene, cleaning, and recycling. Healing will become ordinary.

Unfortunately, healing is still considered extraordinary. The ordinary reaction when facing pain and disease is either to hide or fight— the same responses we have to emotional aggression, and even though no satisfying resolve ever came from such reactions but more suffering. We are caught in a system of reflexes, of habits, of traditions, of things always being done that way, and being caught up with competitiveness, scapegoating, vindictiveness, revenge, and other atavistic reactions reminiscent of vendettas and clan wars, unfinished business from a time long gone. It is thus quite extraordinary to face insult and emotional pain with understanding and compassion—for oneself as well as for others—and to let go of preconditioned reflexes that throw us into a fighting mode. Such extraordinary reactions characterize what it is to be truly human: to respond from a place of respect and compassion, to take care of the poor, the sick, and the weak, and to contribute to the evolution of the human race by actively participating in our own betterment as well as others'.

Healing, at the individual level, is synonymous to evolving and fulfilling one's life purpose. At the community level, healing means integrating and harmonizing a personal level of interaction into better-functioning relationships, evolving into a more significant level of participation for the good of all. At the society level, healing is about being able to take care of a society's members at all levels of existence. All spiritual leaders from the beginning of recorded history, from all creeds, have taught love and compassion as the saving grace for suffering and the healthy growth of the human soul. Isn't it about time that we integrate these principles into the fabric of our social life, especially in the care of the sick and weak, of children and the elderly, of the disenfranchised and disabled. And shouldn't we have such integration be fully reflected in a comprehensive health care system that would include healing?

The whole universe is in a perpetual state of expansion; so are our consciousness and our capacity to evolve and become more human. Nothing can stop that evolution. In the past few years, centers for yoga, meditation, and healing have become a more common sight. Indeed, we nowadays commonly have access to alternative or complementary medical modalities. There are now laws that recognize and protect practitioners of such modalities, as in the states of California and Minnesota where unlicensed practitioners are free to practice their art under the Health Freedom State Bill.[15] These practitioners are now able to work with medical doctors to provide clients with optimal care. Insurance companies are more willing to cover massage therapy, acupuncture, naturopathy, and other popular modalities, as they realize how much money they can save avoiding more expensive allopathic procedures. Also, and especially where access to health freedom is more restricted, informed people adopt to go abroad to seek the care they need—they practice medical tourism, filling classes and workshops in holistic modalities around the world.

To provide healing is an art. Practitioners have studied, trained, and gone through their own healing process. It is much easier to work on someone else than to work on oneself, and once a procedure works on oneself, it has an even greater chance of working on someone else. Healing, like many forms of art, is simple, yet not easy. To be able to differentiate within a health condition the different personal factors involved in making the development of a disease possible, to be able to recognize a meaning and an emotional charge hidden behind the malfunction of a body system according to its location and particular manifestation, takes wisdom and emotional maturity. That maturity is part of the natural evolution of a humanity that will eventually be making medicine more human and healing more ordinary.

There are no sects,
No others,
No you.
Buddha-past,
Buddha-present
Buddha-future,
Are all the same.

Ly Thai Tong (999–1054)[16]

Bibliography

Capra, Fritjof. *The Tao of Physics*. Boulder, CO.: Shambhala Publications, 1975.

———. *The Turning Point*. New York: Bantam New Age Books, 1982.

———. *The Web of Life*. New York: Anchor Books, 1996.

Chang, Stephen. *The Great Tao*. San Francisco: Tao Publishing, 1987.

Chia, Mantak. *Chi Nei Tsang*. Huntington, NY: Healing Tao Books, 1989.

———. *Fusion of the Five Elements*. Huntington, NY: Healing Tao Books, 1989.

Chopra, Deepak. *Quantum Healing*. New York: Bantam Books, 1990.

Connely, Diane M. *The Law of Five Elements*. Columbia, MD: Center for Traditional Acupuncture Inc., 1979.

Feldenkrais, Moshe. *Awareness Through Movement*. San Francisco: Harper Collins, 1972.

Gallo, Fred. *Energy Psychology*. Boca Raton, FL: CRC Press, 1999.

Goleman, Daniel. *Emotional Intelligence*. New York: Bantam Books, 1995.

Hammer, Leon. *Dragon Rises, Red Bird Flies*. Barrytown, NY: Station Hill Press, Inc., 1990.

Kaptchuk, Ted. *The Web That Has No Weaver*. Chicago: Congdon & Weed, 1983.

Mann, Felix. *Acupuncture*. New York: Random House, 1962.

Marin, Gilles. *Healing from Within with Chi Nei Tsang*. Berkeley: North Atlantic Books, 1999.

Murphy, Michael. *The Future of the Body*. Los Angeles: Jeremy Tarcher, Inc., 1992.

Ni, Hua Ching. *I Ching: The Book of Change and the Unchanging Truth*. Santa Monica: Sevenstar Communications Group, 1983.

Nocquet, André. *Présence et Message*. Paris: Guy Trédaniel, edition de la Maisnie, 1975.

Sheldrake, Rupert. *A New Science of Life: The Hypothesis of Morphic Resonance*. Rochester, VT: Park Street Press, 1995.

Stevens, John. *Invincible Warrior*. Boston: Shambhala Publications, 1997.

Tanahashi, Kazuaki. "The story of ideographs," *Aikido Today* magazine, no. 59, Sept./Oct. 1998.

Tokitsu, Kenji. *Miyamoto Musashi*. Boston: Shambhala Publications, 2004.

Yan, Johnson F. *DNA and the I Ching*. Berkeley: North Atlantic Books, 1991.

Yu Huan, Zhang, and Ken Rose. *A Brief History of Chi*. Brookline, MA: Paradigm Publications, 2001.

Zukav, Gary. *The Dancing Wu-Li Masters*. New York: Bantam Book, 1979.

Notes

1 Please read the works of Fritjof Capra, *The Tao of Physics;* Gary Zukav, *The Dancing Wu-Li Masters;* Deepak Chopra, *Quantum Healing;* and Johnson F. Yan, *DNA and the I'Ching.*

2 See *Healing from Within with Chi Nei Tsang,* p. 69.

3 See Kazuaki Tanahashi, "The story of ideographs."

4 Ibid.

5 John Stevens, *Invincible Warrior.*

6 See Chapter 2 of *Healing from Within.*

7 See Johnson F. Yan, *DNA and the I'Ching.*

8 See Hua-Ching Ni, *I Ching: The Book of Changes and the Unchanging Truth.*

9 See Rupert Sheldrake, *A New Science of Life: The Hypothesis of Morphic Resonance.*

10 Norman Cousins, *Anatomy of an Illness,* (New York: W. W. Norton and Co., 1979).

11 Gilles Marin, *Breathing Chi-Kung* CD, Disc 1 track 3, *Healing from Within* Audio Series, 1993.

12 From Walt Whitman, *Leaves of Grass* (New York: Barnes & Noble, 1993).

13 Mantak Chia, *Fusion of the Five Elements.*

14 Spino-Mandibular Equilibration, or SME, is an advanced technique of Chi Nei Tsang involving the use of a mouthpiece to maintain the jaws in a neutral position while working with the general alignment of the body.

15 California State Bill 577 in California, as of 2002.

16 From Burton Raffel, *From the Vietnamese: Ten Centuries of Poetry.*

Index